CHILDREN'S ISSUES, LAWS AND PROGRAMS

PREVENTION OF CHILDHOOD OBESITY: INTERVENTION PROGRAMS

CHILDREN'S ISSUES, LAWS AND PROGRAMS

Additional books in this series can be found on Nova's website under the Series tab.

Additional E-books in this series can be found on Nova's website under the E-books tab.

NUTRITION AND DIET RESEARCH PROGRESS

Additional books in this series can be found on Nova's website under the Series tab.

Additional E-books in this series can be found on Nova's website under the E-books tab.

CHILDREN'S ISSUES, LAWS AND PROGRAMS

PREVENTION OF CHILDHOOD OBESITY: INTERVENTION PROGRAMS

CHRISTINA V. MANCUSO
EDITOR

Library of Congress Cataloging-in-Publication Data

Prevention of childhood obesity : intervention programs / [edited by]
Christina V. Mancuso.
p. cm.
Includes index.
ISBN 978-1-61209-962-0 (hardcover)
1. Obesity in children--Prevention. I. Mancuso, Christina V.
RJ399.C6P744 2011
618.92'398--dc22

2011005837

Published by Nova Science Publishers, Inc. † New York

CONTENTS

PREFACE

As the search for solutions that effectively address childhood obesity continues, organizations and communities across the country are experimenting with innovative strategies and new ways of implementing existing interventions aimed at changing children's environments to prevent obesity. This new book is an overview of the Early Assessment of Programs and Policies to Prevent Childhood Obesity project which identifies and assesses at the local-level programs that have been implemented with apparent success to prevent obesity by improving eating habits and physical activity levels of children. The project is a collaborative effort led by a team from the Robert Wood Johnson Foundation and the Centers for Disease Control and Prevention.

Chapter 1- Early Assessment of Programs and Policies to Prevent Childhood Obesity was a 2-year project to identify and assess local-level programs and policies that have been implemented with apparent success to prevent obesity by improving the eating habits and physical activity levels of children. The project is a collaborative effort led by a team from the Robert Wood Johnson Foundation (RWJF) and the Centers for Disease Control and Prevention (CDC). In both project years, a systematic screening and assessment method identified programs and policies for consideration by an expert panel. Priority was given to initiatives addressing low-income populations and ethnic groups that experience disproportionate childhood obesity rates.

Chapter 2- The Early Assessment of Programs and Policies to Prevent Childhood Obesity was a 2-year project to identify and assess local-level programs and policies to prevent obesity that have been implemented with notable success. The authors focused on promising environmental interventions implemented in community settings intended to improve the eating habits and physical activity levels of children aged 3 to 17 years. They gave priority to programs that addressed low-income populations and ethnic groups that experience disproportionate childhood obesity.

Chapter 3- Early Assessment of Programs and Policies to Prevent Childhood *Obesity* is a 2-year project to identify and assess local-level programs and policies that have been implemented with apparent success to prevent obesity by improving the eating habits and physical activity levels of children aged 3 to 17 years. In each year of the project, a systematic search process identified programs and policies, and then an expert panel suggested further exploration of the most promising programs and policies. Priority was given to programs and policies that addressed low-income populations and ethnic groups with disproportionate childhood obesity.

Chapter 4- Early Assessment of Programs and Policies to Prevent Childhood Obesity was a 2-year project to identify and assess local-level programs and policies that have been implemented with apparent success to prevent obesity by improving the eating habits and physical activity levels of children aged 3 to 17 years. In each year of the project, a systematic search process identified programs and policies, and then an expert panel suggested further exploration of the most promising programs and policies. Priority was given to programs and policies that addressed low-income populations and ethnic groups with disproportionate childhood obesity.

In: Prevention of Childhood Obesity
Editor: Christina V. Mancuso, pp. 1-41
ISBN: 978-1-61209-962-0

Chapter 1

Childcare Initiatives in Afterschool and Daycare Settings

Christina V. Mancuso

Acknowledgments

This project is a collaborative effort led by a team from the Robert Wood Johnson Foundation (RWJF); the Centers for Disease Control and Prevention's (CDC) Division of Nutrition, Physical Activity and Obesity; Division of Adolescent and School Health, Division of Adult and Community Health's Prevention Research Centers Program Office; and the CDC Foundation. The project team is advised by the Funder's Advisory Committee, which includes representatives from the RWJF, the National Institutes for Health, the U.S. Department of Agriculture (USDA), WK Kellogg Foundation, and Kaiser Permanente. ICF Macro, an ICF International Company, serves as the Coordinating Center for the project.

We are appreciative to administrators and staff at the selected childcare initiatives who opened their doors to our project team. Interviews were often lengthy and the openness of the staff enable this report to describe what was learned from the initiatives and assists others who may be developing a new childcare initiative addressing childhood obesity.

I. Introduction

Early Assessment of Programs and Policies to Prevent Childhood Obesity was a 2-year project to identify and assess local-level programs and policies that have been implemented with apparent success to prevent obesity by improving the eating habits and physical activity levels of children. The project is a collaborative effort led by a team from the Robert Wood Johnson Foundation (RWJF) and the Centers for Disease Control and Prevention (CDC). In both project years, a systematic screening and assessment method identified programs and policies for consideration by an expert panel. Priority was given to initiatives addressing low-income populations and ethnic groups that experience disproportionate childhood obesity rates.

Purpose of Systematic Screening and Assessment Method

As the search for solutions that effectively address childhood obesity continues, organizations and communities across the country are experimenting with innovative strategies and new ways of implementing existing interventions aimed at changing children's environments to prevent obesity. The Systematic Screening and Assessment (SSA) Method screens environmental and policy initiatives that show the potential to be effective in controlling childhood obesity.

As part of the SSA Method, evaluability assessments were used to assess the plausibility and feasibility of selected programs and policies that were identified as promising during the search process and selected by the project's expert panel. Evaluability assessment is a process in which evaluators work with program administrators and stakeholders to determine an initiative's readiness for evaluation (Patton, 1997). It involves clarifying goals and program design by specifying the program model, finding out stakeholders' views on the important issues, and exploring program reality (Wholey, 2004). Evaluability assessments can help determine whether a rigorous evaluation study (e.g., an experimental design such as a randomized control trial) is feasible and merited for a particular intervention. As such, they can help avoid premature investment in rigorous evaluation of programs or policies that have not been adequately implemented and allow evaluation resources to be targeted to programs or policies deemed ready for evaluation.

During each year of the 2-year project, focus areas were selected. Initiatives were then identified through a systematic nomination and selection process.

Policy or environmental initiatives implemented in community settings intended to address obesity in children aged 3 to 17 years were considered. Once meeting inclusion and exclusion criteria, initiatives were summarized for the project's expert panel. The expert panel consisted of researchers and evaluators with experience in nutrition, physical activity, and health promotion programs. The expert panel selected initiatives to receive an evaluability assessment based on potential impact, innovativeness, reach to target population, acceptability to stakeholders, feasibility of implementation, and feasibility of adoption, intervention sustainability, generalizability, and staff/organizational capacity. Once an initiative was selected, two site visitors conducted a 2- to 4-day evaluability assessment, which consisted of a document review, travel to conduct interviews and observe the program, drafting a logic model, and summarizing what was learned.

Focus Areas

For both years of the project, the Funder's Advisory Committee identified four thematic areas: (1) childcare programs and policies in afterschool and daycare settings, (2) increasing access to healthier foods, (3) school district local wellness policies and (4) comprehensive school physical activity programs. This report focuses on childcare initiatives in the afterschool and daycare settings. It describes the findings from the 21 evaluability assessments that took place for both years and concludes with lessons learned.

II. Opportunities in Childcare for Obesity Prevention

Childhood overweight has been an increasing problem over the past few decades. Almost 16% of children and adolescents aged 2 to 19 years are overweight based on 2005 to 2006 estimates (Ogden, Carroll, & Flegal, 2008). Overweight children and adolescents are at an increased risk for adverse levels of several cardiovascular disease risk factors compared to normal weight children and adolescents (Freedman, Dietz, Srinivasan, & Berenson, 1999).

Physical Activity

Children who engage in regular physical activity typically have lower levels of body fat (U.S. Department of Health and Human Services, 2008a). In addition to increasing the likelihood of being a healthy weight, regular physical activity provides a multitude of health benefits such as improved cardiorespiratory and muscular fitness, improved bone health, and improved cardiovascular and metabolic health biomarkers (U.S. Department of Health and Human Services, 2008a).

The Department of Health and Human Services' *2008 Physical Activity Guidelines for Americans* (U.S. Department of Health and Human Services, 2008a) are provided for those aged 6 years and older. Guidelines state children aged 6 to 17 years should receive 60 or more minutes of daily physical activity, where most of the 60 minutes should be either moderate or vigorous intensity. These are consistent with National Association for Sport and Physical Education (NASPE) recommendations and achieving *Healthy People 2010* goals (National Association for Sport and Physical Education, 2004; U.S. Department of Health and Human Services, 2000). The *Physical Activity Guidelines* also recommend muscle- and bone-strengthening exercises at least 3 days per week, which should be part of the 60 or more minutes. It is recommended that physical activity be age-appropriate, enjoyable, and varied. Unstructured play can also help meet recommendations. However, as children age, structured activity becomes a more appropriate way to be physically active. Physical activity is also recommended for children with disabilities (U.S. Department of Health and Human Services, 2008b). Afterschool initiatives are an ideal setting to increase physical activity levels because time spent in physical activity during the school day may not reach recommended levels (Nader, 2003; McKenzie et al., 1995).

While the *2008 Physical Activity Guidelines* do not have recommendations for children under age 6 years, other recommendations exist. The American Academy of Pediatrics recommends providing a 15 to 20 minutes structured activity combined with 30 minutes of free play for younger children (Committee on Sports Medicine and Fitness and Committee on School Health, 2001) and NASPE recommends preschoolers participate in at least 60 minutes of structured and at least 60 minutes of unstructured physical activity per day (National Association for Sport and Physical Education, 2002). Because of the length of time children often spend in daycare, this setting is ideal for offering time for children to be engaged in physical activity.

Nutrition

In addition to lack of physical activity, poor diet is a contributor to obesity. Afterschool and daycare initiatives may be able to address nutrition by serving healthy snacks and meals to children. The *2005 Dietary Guidelines*, which provide dietary recommendations for Americans older than age 2 (U.S. Department of Health and Human Services & U.S. Department of Agriculture, 2005) can be used to guide nutritional standards in afterschool or daycare programs.

Afterschool and daycare initiatives frequently face challenges to providing healthy foods that meet the *Dietary Guidelines*. These may include financial constraints and other competing priorities, inconvenience, or not placing high value on offering healthier options. Another issue afterschool and daycare settings confront is whether to permit children to bring their own snacks and beverages because these foods may be unhealthy.

Afterschool Initiatives

Afterschool initiatives offer an avenue to increase participation in moderate to vigorous physical activity (MVPA), provide a healthy snack, and educate youth on healthy eating. A large proportion of children are enrolled in some form of afterschool care. As of 2005, 40% of students in kindergarten through eighth grade were enrolled in afterschool care at least once per week (Carver & Iruka, 2006).

There is evidence that afterschool initiatives can successfully address physical activity and nutrition. One 10-month study of an afterschool physical activity program found beneficial changes in body composition and cardiovascular fitness in 8- to 12-year-old African American girls (Barbeau et al., 2007). In Texas, the CATCH (Coordinated Approach to Child Health) program was adapted to an afterschool program, CATCH Kids Club (CKC), which aimed to increase MVPA in 16 afterschool programs; children significantly increased their levels of MVPA during the 6-month study period compared to the control group (Kelder et al., 2005). The FitKid project, an 8-month afterschool program, offered third-grade students a healthy snack following the United States Department of Agriculture's (USDA) National School Lunch Program afterschool snack guidelines and an 80-minutes period that included 40 minutes of continuous MVPA. Results revealed a relative reduction in percentage of body fat compared to a control group (Yin et al., 2005a; 2005b).

Daycare Initiatives

Daycare centers are another setting to focus efforts on addressing childhood obesity, particularly because young children may spend a large amount of time in daycare centers where there is potential to influence physical activity and food consumption. There are more then 118,000 daycare centers in the United States, and approximately 18% of children are younger than age 5 of employed mothers are enrolled in daycare (National Association of Child Care Resource & Referral Agencies, 2008). Children in this age group (2 to 5 years) are at risk for being obese. In the 2 to 5-year age group, about 12% of children are obese, with 24.4% classified as overweight (Ogden et al., 2008).

Good feeding and eating experiences early in life shape dietary preferences and may affect the quality of nutrition throughout childhood (Fuller, Keller, Olson, & Plymale, 2005). Because children develop food and nutrition-related attitudes during the preschool years (Fuller et al., 2005), and the daycare setting provides a venue in which to teach nutrition, offer nutritious foods, provide opportunities to try new foods, and there is potential for shaping behaviors in later life.

There is limited evidence describing the nutritional quality of foods served and activity levels in daycare settings (Story, Kaphingst, & French, 2006). However, evidence is available from those daycare programs that participate in the USDA's Child and Adult Care Food Program (CACFP) that meals and snacks being served are high in fat, saturated fat, and lacking fruits and vegetables (U.S. Department of Agriculture, 2008; Story et al., 2006). Story and colleagues (Story et al., 2006) recommend CACFP comply with the U.S. *Dietary Guidelines*.

Adequate physical activity time during daycare hours is also essential. Prior research has demonstrated that physical activity levels can range from 4.4. to 10.2 minutes of MVPA per hour during the preschool day (Pate, Pfeiffer, Trost, Ziegler, & Dowda, 2004). Institutional policies and practices that offer greater opportunities for physical activity may meet this standard through policies that require children to spend 60 minutes in structured play while also offering time for unstructured play.

Because many children spend time in afterschool and daycare settings where there is opportunity to offer nutritious meals/snacks and MVPA, afterschool and day care settings were selected for the Early Assessment project. Results from the evaluability assessments have the potential to fill some research gaps as well as identify promising practices that can be shared with the field. For afterschool and daycare initiatives, these include (1) understanding how to engage children in MVPA, (2) identifying strategies to engage parents in their child's diet and physical activity habits, and (3) identifying ways to educate parents on nutrition and physical activity during the brief window of opportunity when the parents come to pick up their child.

III. METHODS

Nomination of Programs and Policies

The project team solicited nominations for afterschool and daycare initiatives in spring 2007 for year 1 and spring/summer 2008 for year 2. Postings were put on a variety of listservs (e.g., CDC's Chronic Disease Nutrition listserv), and contacts were made with organizations familiar with afterschool or daycare initiatives (e.g., YMCA).

For both project years, nominated programs and policies were eligible for inclusion in the project if they were an environmental program or policy taking place in an afterschool or daycare setting that were suitable for the United States (i.e., either taking place in the United States or in a developed country), being implemented during the scheduled time evaluability assessments, had a primary goal to address nutrition or physical activity, had not previously been evaluated, and were not a strict replication of an evidence-based model.

During year 1, a total of 81 afterschool and daycare initiatives were nominated, 34 met inclusion criteria, and 25 were summarized for the expert panel. Nine initiatives met the criteria for inclusion, but were not summarized for several reasons (e.g., contact could not be made with the program nominator to complete a program summary after multiple attempts before the deadline, or the deadline had passed before the program nomination was received).

During year 2, 86 afterschool and daycare initiatives were nominated, 27 met eligibility criteria, and 25 were summarized for the expert panel. Two were not summarized because contact could not be made with the person who nominated the initiative before the deadline.

Criteria and Selection of Programs and Policies for Evaluability Assessments

The expert panel used the following criteria to select initiatives for evaluability assessment: potential impact, innovativeness, reach to target population, acceptability to stakeholders, feasibility of implementation, and feasibility of adoption, intervention sustainability, generalizability, and staff/organizational capacity. See Appendix A for a detailed description of each criterion. For both years, the expert panel reviewed and rated each summarized initiative using an online survey tool followed by in-person recommendations on which initiatives should receive an evaluability assessment. For year 1, 10 of the 25 summarized afterschool and daycare initiatives were selected for evaluability assessments: 7 afterschool and 3 daycare initiatives. Eight afterschool and four daycare initiatives were selected for year 2. One evaluability assessment was not conducted on one of the selected afterschool initiatives in year 2 because initial follow-up revealed the program was very different from how it was originally presented. Therefore, seven afterschool initiatives were visited in year 2.

Afterschool and Daycare Evaluability Assessments

Evaluability assessments consisted of two trained site visitors (1) reviewing background documents for their initiative, (2) drafting a logic model to graphically describe the initiative's activities, desired outcomes, and goals, (3) traveling to the location of the initiative to observe the initiative in progress and conduct interviews with staff and stakeholders to assess development, implementation, funding, data collection, and evaluation capacity. During year 1, the afterschool evaluability assessments took place in Texas, Wisconsin, Ohio, Kentucky, North Carolina, Pennsylvania, and New York. Two daycare evaluability assessments occurred in New York and one in North Carolina. During year 2, three afterschool evaluability assessments took place in California and one each in Colorado, Oklahoma, Nebraska, Missouri, and Ohio. The daycare initiatives were located in Ohio, North Carolina, and the Virginia/Washington, DC area. Each year, after the evaluability assessments took place, the project team and expert panel reviewed the findings from the evaluability assessments to discuss their promise and readiness for rigorous evaluation.

Data Analysis

For each evaluability assessment, site visitors wrote summary reports describing what was learned during the site visit. The summary reports served as the primary data source for this report. Common themes were extracted from the site visit reports using ATLAS.ti (Scientific Software Development GmbH, 2008) a qualitative analysis program. Prior to coding, two coders conducted test runs of site visit reports to ensure reliability. Discrepancies between coders were discussed and resolved. Coding for the childcare thematic area was carried out by an independent coder. Codes fell into larger themes, such as plausibility, feasibility, program/policy components, and staff capacity. Site visitors reviewed coding results to ensure coders accurately interpreted the information. A secondary data source for this report includes expert panel members' recommendations regarding the initiatives.

IV. RESULTS

Goals and Anticipated Outcomes of the Afterschool and Daycare Initiatives

The most common goals outlined by the initiatives were increasing physical activity and fitness levels, improving nutritional intake during the time children were enrolled in the program, gaining parental buy-in, and incorporating staff wellness components. The most common end-goal was to impact childhood obesity, whether through increased physical activity, improved nutrition, or both.

Target Audience

All afterschool initiatives targeted children of elementary school age, while two also included children as young as kindergarten. Nine afterschool programs included parents as a target audience and four also included staff as a target audience. One of the Early Assessment project's goals was to focus on initiatives serving minority populations. Within our sample, six afterschool initiatives targeted Latinos, African Americans, or Native American Indians. While other programs did not specify a particular race/ethnic group, they targeted urban youth or urban and suburban youth, and were reaching high minority populations. Additionally, all afterschool programs served children from economically disadvantaged groups; however, 10 focused specifically on low socioeconomic status (SES) families.

The daycare initiatives targeted all children enrolled in the daycare center(s), as well as parents. All daycare initiatives, with one exception, also included staff as a target audience. In addition, all daycare initiative were either serving children of regardless of their SES status or specifically targeting low SES children and families. One daycare program specifically targeted ZIP codes where there were higher rates of obesity. Two other daycare programs reached urban and rural children throughout their community.

Reach

Reach varied for afterschool initiatives; the range was 1 to 111 sites, with a median of 20 sites. Afterschool initiatives reported a wide range for the total number of children being reached; 11 children to approximately 5,500, with a median of 1,100 (two programs did not report the number of children being reached). Programs reaching many children across several sites tended to be YMCA-based programs. Daycare initiatives also varied in how many centers they were reaching; 3 to more than 2,000, with a median of 52 sites (two did not report the number of sites). The range for number of children being reached was 300 to 300,000, with a median of 1,820 children.

Afterschool/Daycare Logic Model

As part of each evaluability assessment, program/policy administrators, stakeholders, and staff worked with the site visitors to tailor a logic model to their initiative based on a standard template. Appendix B provides an example logic model with appropriate information entered into each box. The logic models for each initiative in the childcare setting were reviewed for commonalities and differences. This section discusses two components of the logic model: (1) Inputs and (2) Activities and Outputs.

Inputs

The findings relevant to the Inputs section of the logic model clustered in five main areas: staffing, resources, funding, target audience, and nutrition and/or physical activity guidelines.

Staffing

Interviewees frequently explained that a dedicated and knowledgeable staff was important to keeping the program running. There are several examples of afterschool and daycare initiatives where administrators hired staff with knowledge and skills that would benefit their program. Examples include experience in teaching physical education, health promotion program planning, or implementing programs on a large scale. Staff at one afterschool program was able to develop, with the help of the physical education instructors on staff, a curriculum with 70 lesson plans to maintain children's interest in physical activity. A second example includes a manager with experience in health promotion planning who helped design and implement an afterschool program that reached approximately 1,400 students and then designed an evaluation.

High levels of staff turnover is a common challenge within the childcare industry (Center for the Childcare Workforce, 2004). The initiatives that received an evaluability assessment echoed this. High turnover may lead to problems with program fidelity because staff may not be present for trainings if they are held only once or at pre-specified intervals. Several initiatives addressed this issue by holding initial trainings when staff first started, instead of at pre-specified intervals, and also held frequent staff trainings that allowed staff to maintain their programmatic knowledge.

Various staff structures and chains of command existed in the afterschool programs. In many cases, a centrally located, high-level administrative staff designed the program, which was then implemented by part-time afterschool instructors, employed by the agency that developed the program, at multiple locations throughout the program's catchment area. For example, administrators at a county YMCA developed a program and had their own afterschool instructors implement the program in various locations throughout the county. Another model is an afterschool program developed by a central team of administrators (e.g., a university professor and health department personnel) where part-time afterschool instructors were trained to implement the program. The part-time afterschool instructors were employees of other agencies with already existing afterschool programs, such as Boys and Girls Club and the YMCA.

Resources

Community partnerships are an example of the resources many initiatives relied upon. Community partnerships provided social support for the program and helped programs meet their objectives. Community support ranged from supplemental funding to social marketing to donating time. One example is an afterschool program receiving community support in the form of local chefs volunteering their time to demonstrate how to prepare healthy meals during afterschool sessions on a regular basis. Children observed the chef and ate appropriate portions immediately after the chef finished.

Another community resource is evaluators and researchers from local universities or local health departments. Three afterschool programs had the assistance of a faculty member employed at a nearby university. One program used this collaboration to have the faculty member conduct a program evaluation on implementing the program. A second afterschool program had university faculty design and develop a program implementation strategy within the afterschool setting. And the third afterschool program with university faculty had their researcher intimately involved with curriculum development, implementation, and evaluation. One afterschool program serves as a good example of enlisting the help of an evaluator from a local health department. This evaluator provided technical assistance on program implementation and encouraged the program developers to consider evaluation.

Funding

Funding for the afterschool and daycare initiatives varied in amount and type. Funding came from Federal (e.g., CDC, USDA's Food Stamp Nutrition Education Program), State, and private dollars (e.g., local medical center), as well as from partner organizations and philanthropic foundations. Those program needs that were not met by such mechanisms were met by offering services on a fee-based model.

Many afterschool initiatives relied on several funding sources; the reported number of sources ranged from 2 to 18. Sites were also asked to provide the estimated costs of their initiative, however, these were challenging to ascertain. Eight afterschool programs reported dollar amounts ranging from approximately $15,000 to $700,000. It is not possible to determine if these are start-up or annual operational costs; many provided a listing of the grants and donations they received. Other initiatives were unable to provide dollar amounts because their afterschool program was one part of a larger grant or staff worked on the afterschool program but also had additional responsibilities not related to the afterschool program. Programs that tended to have many funding sources or higher funding amounts typically had a larger reach, but not always. Examples include having 18 funding sources reaching more than 2,500 children across 16 schools or having funding more than $650,000 and reaching more than 110 schools. An example of a program that seems more costly is a program with funding of approximately $250,000 per year with a reach of slightly less than 100 children. However, this funding includes staff salaries and also efforts that went to non-afterschool programming.

Daycare initiatives reported from 2 to 13 funding sources, with one exception. The exception is a daycare program reporting zero outside funding sources. After a small start-up grant of $4,000 was obtained, the program continued as a line item in the annual budget. Funding amounts ranged from $4,000 up to $1.4 million. Daycare initiatives often blended funding sources to implement their programs; for example, one daycare program received $500,000 for the first year of implementation and $1.2 million for the second year from a federal source, and matched these funds with state health department dollars of $95,000 per year. While the daycare policy did not require funding, childcare staff time was necessary to make changes in food purchasing habits or obtain additional equipment to ensure foods provided adhered to the policy and there was adequate equipment to meet physical activity regulations. The Sports, Play, and Active Recreation for Kids (SPARK) program, which is widely used but not mandated by the daycare policy, requires an annual purchase. The reported amount for the 2007 to 2008 fiscal year was $1.4 million for SPARK, which the city health department purchased. Programs and policies with higher funding amounts had larger reach than those with lower funding amounts.

Use of Physical Activity and Nutrition Guidelines

Several initiatives use physical activity and nutrition guidelines from various sources. The following physical activity guidelines were reportedly used: NASPE (for two daycare initiatives), and CANFIT (one afterschool initiative) (National Association for Sport and Physical Education, 2002; California After School Resource Center, 2006). Several initiatives developed their own rules for length of time children should be engaged in physical activity and several also sought guidance from physical education instructors.

Seven afterschool and daycare initiatives were following at least one of the following guidelines: the USDA Child Adult Care Feeding Program, the *2005 Dietary Guidelines for Americans*, Institute of Medicine (IOM) guidelines for snack foods, *Healthy People 2010* nutrition objectives, and CANFIT nutrition guidelines. (U.S. Department of Health and Human Services & U.S. Department of Agriculture, 2005; Committee on Nutrition Standards for Foods in Schools Food and Nutrition Board, 2007; U.S. Department of Health and Human Services, 2000; Tides Center, 2009).

While several programs reported specific guidelines they were following, other programs also ensured their program or policy components were grounded in scientific evidence. Examples of documents that programs referred to include *Bright Futures in Practice: Nutrition, Bright Futures in Practice: Physical Activity, Institute of Medicine Report: Preventing Childhood Obesity, Health in the Balance* (Story, Holt, & Sofka, 2002; Patrick, Spear, Holt, & Sofka, 2001; Committee on Prevention of Obesity in Children and Youth, 2005). Some initiatives also conducted scientific literature reviews to ensure they had an understanding of physical activity and nutrition for their age group and target audience.

Activities and Outputs

Common Program and Policy Activities

General program activities, most of which are necessary for program maintenance and sustainability, tended to include activities in the following categories: enrollment of children into the program; staff training, staff meetings and professional development; parental engagement (often via newsletters or information sent home with children); curriculum revision; and community partnership-building activities. The majority of initiatives did not list evaluation as a priority, with the exception of one program which included grant writing and accompanying evaluation tasks as a primary activity. See Appendix C for detailed program and policy components.

Physical Activity and Nutrition Activities

All initiatives attempted to increase physical activity and physical fitness levels, and most incorporated nutrition components. Some initiatives ensured that moderate to vigorous physical activity took place five days a week, while others tried to engage children in any intensity of physical activity fewer days of the week.

With one exception, every initiative included in this project addressed nutrition by either serving healthier snacks or by offering nutrition education. Most reported improving offerings to provide healthier snacks and meals; but four programs only provided nutrition education and did not change the meal or snack provided. The most common reason was it was not in their purview to do so; food service was under the direction of others, rendering control impossible. However, two programs reported contacting food service staff to improve snack offerings, but this was not successful for both programs.

Parental Engagement Activities

Afterschool program and policy developers designed a range of strategies to involve parents. Parental involvement was achieved by holding family nights to engage in physical activity, family nights with cooking demonstrations and dinner, and grocery shopping trips with a registered dietician to plan family meals. Other examples include providing information to parents through newsletters, a handbook, and brochures with health messages. One afterschool program developed parent pledges which were written promises to eat healthier and to engage in physical activity. Pledges were signed by the parents and parents were asked to post the top portion of the pledge to their refrigerator as a reminder. Another afterschool program offered events for entire families so all could participate in activities with all of their children.

All daycare initiatives took steps to involve parents. Parental engagement ranged from providing information to offering trainings for parents. For example, one program gave children a take home sheet to notify parents of the lesson taught to the child with a recipe included. The daycare policy asked daycare centers to distribute fliers to parents and educate parents on the policy components. In addition, trainings for parents were held to gain parental support for the policy by educating parents on healthier food items that were permitted to be sent with their child to daycare.

Staff Wellness Activities

Staff wellness components were also common, especially in daycare initiatives. Six out of seven daycare initiatives had a staff wellness component such as nutrition education for staff, requiring staff to engage in physical activity with the children, and teaching staff the importance of modeling healthy behaviors. Four afterschool initiatives had formal staff wellness components that restricted beverages that the staff could consume in front of the children or required staff to participate in the physical activity time with the children.

Additional Activities

In addition to addressing physical activity and nutrition, there are several examples of initiatives incorporating additional activities. Three initiatives addressed the importance of limiting television viewing and video time. Three initiatives integrated components such as health literacy and commitment to a healthy lifestyle through education. Another afterschool program that focused on Native Americans taught traditional Indian games.

Evaluation Activities

Evaluating childcare initiatives aiming to reduce obesity can help fill evidence gaps for the afterschool and daycare settings. The vast majority of the selected initiatives appear promising. While it is uncertain if they will impact body mass index (BMI), they can contribute to increasing healthy eating behaviors through nutrition education and offering healthier snacks and addressing physical activity by engaging children in 60 minutes of physical activity five days per week.

Devoting time and effort to evaluation is often challenging, but some initiatives either engaged in process evaluation or were in planning stages of an outcome evaluation. Those engaging in process evaluation were collecting relevant data. For example, one afterschool initiative was evaluating staff trainings to determine level of knowledge gained and whether or not program components were being implemented properly. Four initiatives were either collecting data or had plans to collect data to measure fitness levels, height and weight to calculate BMI, or use Fitnessgram, which are assessments on aerobic capacity, body composition, muscle strength, endurance, and flexibility (Welk & Meredith, 2008). These data could be a part of an outcome evaluation. Most initiatives were not actively evaluating their program or policy. The primary reason for this was funding was typically reserved for staff salaries and meeting the needs of the program (e.g., food costs) with little remaining for evaluation.

V. Discussion

Plausibility

Afterschool and daycare initiatives are important settings to address childhood obesity because they can affect children's eating habits and physical activity levels on a daily basis. The goals of the afterschool and daycare initiatives—to improve children's eating habits and increase physical activity levels to reduce childhood obesity—are plausible because of the initiatives' concerted efforts to address nutrition, physical activity, and other components related to healthy living.

We found many examples of initiatives grounding their program or policy in existing science. Program or policy developers consulted existing literature, experts, and resources to guide their initiative. Initiatives were reported plausible at reducing obesity by ensuring adequate physical activity was taking place, focusing on fruit and vegetable intake, low-fat dairy consumption, reducing television viewing time, and more. Additionally, the outreach to staff and parents increase plausibility by staff modeling healthy behaviors and parents being knowledgeable of program components, adhering to policy guidelines, or modeling healthy behaviors themselves.

Because of their sound approach to addressing nutrition and physical activity and their strong management, it is plausible short- and long-term outcomes will be achieved with faithful implementation. Afterschool initiatives have the ability to help children meet physical activity recommendations and to a somewhat lesser extent also affect children's eating habits. Daycare initiatives have the ability to address physical activity and children's eating habits because of the amount of time children frequently spend while in daycare. Both settings can address childhood obesity via physical activity and nutrition, and along with a coordinated approach by the community, parents, and schools, may impact BMI over the long term.

Feasibility of Implementation

Feasibility of implementation, or the likelihood the initiative will be implemented with fidelity, is likely for many of the initiatives with clearly outlined goals, strong leadership, success with obtaining funding, and ensuring trained staff. Initiatives also reported strong stakeholder support, institutionalization of the program, and strong infrastructure, which all further increase the likelihood of feasibility of full implementation.

Feasibility of Adoption

Feasibility of similar sites to adopt the intervention exists because most initiatives considered the audience when designing their program or policy. Most initiatives either tailored their program to low SES children and families, or offered their program in low SES communities. As described above, some initiatives offered family events with free dinners to educate parents on healthy eating and physical activity or offered the program at little to no cost to families. Age-appropriate lessons were also researched and offered as appropriate. Initiatives with similar objectives can use these initiatives as role models when determining which curriculum to follow.

VI. Key Lessons Learned

While each childcare program serves a unique population and thus faces a unique set of challenges and opportunities, several potential barriers to success were found across many initiatives.

Challenges to Offering Physical Activity Opportunities and Engaging Children

As increasing physical activity is included in all program and policy objectives, difficulties in providing or engaging children in the activity can present a major obstacle to meeting expected outcomes. The programs visited had laudable goals for the time devoted to physical activity. However, even within a framework that provides ample time, challenges remain.

Several examples exist where children were bored or did not understand the physical activity they were to be participating in. Many afterschool programs found that children were easily bored if the same activity was frequently offered, and so they provided a range of play activities to stimulate children's interest in being physically active. Multiple games (gathered from various curricula, Web sites, and program staff's imaginations) were played, and children were exposed to various sports as well. One daycare program noticed that some physical activity games were too difficult for young children and modified them with the assistance of early childhood specialists.

When children did not have the desire to participate in physical activity, some initiatives addressed this by requiring staff to participate in the physical activity with the children and model the behavior, and by making a dedicated effort to ensure that children learned to perceive physical activity as fun, not as a chore, by offering varied fun activities suitable for many fitness levels. An example of this was an afterschool program that allowed children to opt out of organized play activities and instead walk around a track.

Challenges to Providing Healthier Snacks

Providing healthier snacks to children was seen as an opportunity by many initiatives, not only as a way for children to consume fruits and vegetables and to limit consumption of less healthy food, but also to increase children's exposure to new healthy foods, countering neophobia and prompting children to ask their parents to purchase healthy options for home.

A challenge specific to some afterschool initiatives is the lack of control over the snacks that are served. Snacks may be under the purview of the school or may be surplus foods leftover from lunch. As a result, snacks may or may not follow any sort of nutritional guidelines. One afterschool program addressed this by partnering with a local distributer to offer low-cost fresh fruit and vegetables for snacks. Another afterschool program experiencing this issue devised two strategies. First, program administrators contacted the food service coordinators, spoke with them about their concerns, and provided suggestions for low-cost, healthier snacks. This approach was reported to be only somewhat successful because food service personnel also faced limitations in what they were able to purchase. Second, program staff made sure to include a nutrition education piece every day, regardless of snack content, in the hope that children would remember a nutrition message.

Childcare initiatives often wished to introduce different or exotic fruits and vegetables to children to increase exposure to new and different foods. One afterschool initiative included a component to expose children to new foods and reported mixed success. When the activities were first offered, children were highly reluctant to try new foods, and parents were wary of any attempts to encourage their children to try new foods. However, the initiative made multiple and varied attempts to present children with new food items in appealing ways.

Challenges to Parental Involvement

Many childcare initiatives reported that engaging parents is challenging. Many parents are unable to take time away from their home life with their children to meet with childcare staff or to participate in program activities—parents often need to quickly pick up their child and continue on with their daily routine. Several afterschool initiatives developed tactics to engage parents during other times of the week, such as the weekend, or offered family nights where the whole family was welcome and dinner was provided. These were not always reported to be highly attended, however, one program did report after offering family night (dinner provided and physical activity time at a local YMCA) twice, the attendance increased greatly. They believed word spread that it was a fun night for families.

Because afterschool programs host children for a small portion of the day, parental engagement is one avenue in which an afterschool program can affect the home environment. By educating parents on the activities of the program, the family is aware of the nutrition education and physical activity their child is receiving and can possibly reinforce some activities outside of program hours.

Another challenge with parental involvement is time in an afterschool program is frequently viewed less as a time for engaging in nutrition education and physical activity and more as a safe and friendly place for children to be watched while their parents are at work. Even among parents who view afterschool care as an educational and enrichment environment, other priorities may take precedence over physical activity and nutrition. For example, afterschool programs frequently reported that homework help was the most desired afterschool activity parents wished for and requested technical assistance with "making the case" for physical activity and nutrition education. Childcare initiatives wishing to involve parents may wish to attempt similar tactics as these initiatives used, such as providing information on what their child is learning, offering recipe ideas, and holding trainings for parents to educate them on what their child will be exposed to during time in the program.

Challenges to Program Fidelity

One particularly delicate challenge for site visitors to address was variation in program fidelity. Some program components, while perceived as fully implemented by program administrators, were viewed by staff working with children more as aspirational goals than required activities.

A clear logic model can assist programs in monitoring program implementation and fidelity. When gaps occur between what is planned and implemented, program administrators can offer additional trainings and education to assist staff or revisit the program design if the challenges to full implementation are more extensive than anticipated during program design. Such events can provide an opportunity to both support staff and to continually improve and refine the program. While a logic model is useful throughout the life of a program, it is particularly useful during the early stages of implementation to identify potential problem areas with fidelity. Creating a logic model may aid future afterschool and daycare initiatives outline desired activities and the importance of these activities for reaching short- and long-term outcomes; this may help identify potential problems with fidelity.

Curricula and Other Resources

Another challenge the initiatives faced and excelled at was determining which curriculum to use or if a new curriculum should be developed. The initiatives either used established curricula, created a new one from scratch, or blended established curricula with their own ideas. This is perhaps the most noteworthy aspect of the initiatives that received an evaluability assessment—their commitment to researching what was best for their target audience and coming up with the best solution.

Resources on childcare initiatives are available. Many are inexpensive or available at no cost:

- Resources on Afterschool: http://www.afterschoolresources.org
- Afterschool Alliance: http://www.afterschoolalliance.org/
- YMCA Programs for Child Care: http://www.ymca.net/programs/programs_for child_care.html

Challenges to Code Compliance (Daycare Policy Only)

A reported challenge specific to the daycare policy is how to enforce code compliance. Staff that would typically be responsible for ensuring compliance are often overburdened with other responsibilities. However, specific daycare sites that were visited stated that the policy enabled them to educate parents and provide guidelines on what children should be eating and what food items parents are permitted to send with their child each day. Therefore, while efforts to find feasible ways to enforce compliance are currently underway, daycare centers are able to explain to parents there is a new policy that the daycare center and parents must follow, which helps enforce compliance. As other cities and states develop similar daycare regulations, enforcing compliance will likely present an ongoing challenge. Hopefully in the near future there will be a model to replicate.

Partnerships and Stakeholders

Creating partnerships and collaborating with pertinent stakeholders is another arena in which the selected initiatives excelled. For example, some initiatives collaborated with local health departments because they did not have the expertise of a nutritionist on staff and others collaborated with local universities to assist with evaluating their initiative and obtaining content expertise in physical activity or nutrition. Building such partnerships and collaborations helps entrench the program in the community and increases awareness and sustainability due to increased interest. Other initiatives may want to follow this example and partner with a local or state health department for assistance or collaborate with local universities, which may have faculty with the appropriate content expertise and could lead an evaluation effort.

VII. Conclusion

The Early Assessment of Programs and Policies to Prevent Childhood Obesity project aimed to discover community-level initiatives that were addressing childhood obesity in afterschool and daycare settings. Because of their reach, programs or policies in these settings have great potential for childhood obesity prevention and control. However, practice-based evidence is needed to determine the core components necessary to effectively improve physical activity levels and nutrition in these settings. This report highlights several noteworthy initiatives that are exposing large numbers of children to healthier eating and physical activity opportunities.

Appendix A. Description of Selection Criteria

Selection Criteria

Potential Impact. The intervention appears to have potential for impact on the social or physical environment pertinent to healthy eating and active living—and ultimately on the target individual behaviors. Potential impact is assessed based on the intervention's conceptual logic and other pertinent characteristics such as intensity and duration. Estimate of impact is based on "face value," program documents, and brief expert input from funding organization staff and contractors, and other experts who know the intervention but are independent from it.

Innovativeness. Intervention is new or different or a significant variation on an existing promising intervention. Emphasis on innovativeness may be mitigated if the intervention represents a type or category of intervention that is prevalent in the field and/or of particular interest to the Foundation and collaborating organizations.

Reach to Target Population. The likelihood or actual evidence that the intervention will achieve participation (and even retention and completion) by the target population (i.e., approximately what percentage of the target population is likely to or actually does participate in or is "reached" in some other way by the intervention).

Acceptability to Stakeholders. The potential or actual evidence that the intervention is acceptable and even attractive to pertinent collaborators, gatekeepers, and other necessary groups such as schools, businesses, government agencies, grassroots groups, etc.

Feasibility of Implementation. The likelihood that the intervention as designed can be implemented fully given the clarity of its goals, objectives and strategies; complexity and leadership requirements; financial and other costs; and training and supervision requirements. If evidence exists regarding program implementation, then the extent to which the intervention "on paper" has been fully and faithfully implemented and the degree of difficulty in achieving implementation.

Feasibility of Adoption. The potential for similar sites/entities to adopt the intervention.

Intervention Sustainability. The likelihood that the intervention can continue over time without special resources or extraordinary leadership.

Generalizability. The degree to which the intervention demonstrates or has potential to be adapted for other populations and settings.

Staff/Organizational Capacity. Sponsoring organization and staff have the capacity to participate fully in a brief assessment, learn from it, and further develop the intervention.

Appendix B. Logic Model

Problem Statement

A healthy diet and adequate physical activity contribute to obesity prevention. After school and daycare programs are vehicles in which to teach and engage children in the benefits of healthier eating and increased physical activity.

INPUTS

Program/Policy Team

- Program/policy developers
- Managers
- Program/policy staff
- Stakeholders
- Evaluators
- Other stakeholders

Resources

- Program Curriculum:
  - Nutrition Curriculum
  - Physical activity (PA) Curriculum
- Nutrition Guidelines
- PA Guidelines
- Funding
- Partnerships
- Obtain the necessary equipment

ACTIVITIES

General Program/Policy

- Obtain informed consent from parents for child to participate
- Establish guidelines/policies to follow
- Trainings held (train-the-trainer model)
- Train staff about program and curricula

Nutrition:

- Children, parents, and/or staff receive nutrition education
- Food service staff receive appropriate training in nutrition
- Other staff receive appropriate training in nutrition
- Healthier snacks and beverages served
- Staff actions to keep program attractive

Physical Activity

- At least XY% of physical activity time is dedicated to MVPA according to the program protocol
- Staff receive appropriate training:
  - in physical activity education
  - how to keep program attractive
  - activities are supervised/ organized

Activities planned (or part of the program design), but not currently implemented

OUTPUTS

General Program/Policy

- Continued participation of those enrolled
- Parents report satisfaction
- Staff report satisfaction

Nutrition

- Children consume healthier snacks and beverages during program hours
- Increased nutrition knowledge for children, parents, and/or staff

Physical Activity

- Children engage in more MVPA during PA time during program hours

SHORT-TERM OUTCOMES (~ 1 to 3 years)

General Program/ Policy

- Program enrollment maintained or increased

Nutrition

- Improved nutrition habits of children inside and outside of program hours

Physical Activity:

- Children engage in the recommended standard of 60 minutes of PA most or all days of the week[1]

INTERMEDIATE OUTCOMES (~ 3 to 5 years)

General Program/ Policy

- Maintenance or increase in program enrollment/ number of locations that implement the program
- Trainings for new locations to implement program

Nutrition

- Continued improvement in nutrition habits of children

Physical Activity

- Children engage in the recommended standard of 60 minutes of PA most or all days of the week[1]

LONG-TERM OUTCOMES (~ 4 to 6 years)

General Program/ Policy

- Program growth through additional locations implementing program

Nutrition

- Maintenance or improvement in eating habits

Physical Activity

- Children engage in the recommended standard of 60 minutes of PA most or all days of the week[1]

GOAL

Contribute to improvement in the eating habits and physical activity levels of youth in after school or daycare programs

Data source to document accomplishment

Outputs:

- Nutrition ed curriculum
- Daily menus
- Number of brochures sent to parents regarding program
- Training sign-in sheets for staff
- Program enrollment (children)
- Number of trainees

Short-term outcomes:

- Pre- and Post- data regarding nutrition knowledge
- Pre- and Post- data regarding physical activity levels
- Pre- and Post- MVPA participation
- Program participation
- Pre- and Post- data regarding level of satisfaction of program (children, staff, and parents)
- Increased funding for additional sites to implement program

Intermediate outcomes:

- Food recall diaries or some other data on eating habits
- Physical activity levels of children
- Program enrollment/number of locations implementing program
- Amount of funding for program implementation

Long-term outcomes:

- Eating habits of children
- Physical activity levels of children
- Number of sites implementing program

[1] USDA. (2005). Physical Activity. *Dietary Guidelines for Americans*, 2005.

Appendix C. Common Program/ Policy Components

			AFTERSCHOOL INITIATIVES				
Location	**Physical Activity**	**Nutrition**	**Duration**	**Other**	**Plausibility**	**Feasibility**	**Potential Impact**
Midwest	Draw destination to "walk" to/PA 4x/week. Any PA qualified of any degree of intensity.	Any sort of nutrition activity; "healthier snacks" encouraged; healthier was not defined.	2 sites visited, 1 implemented over 6 weeks, other over 5 weeks.		Program is based on a plausible theory: increased physical activity and healthier eating will lead to reduction in obesity. Plausibility of program could be increased through increasing intensity of PA and including a stronger nutrition component.	Program feasible because of flexible implementation approach.	The duration (5to6 weeks) of the program may limit its potential impact. Perhaps with a longer duration and more intense PA, potential impact will increase.
Midwest	PA time; focus on football.	Program guide includes Healthy Snack section.	NA		Plausible program can lead to obesity prevention, however, due to limited time children exposed to program, other environmental, policy and behavioral interventions need to occur concurrently.	Model is sound and focused on capacity building of a nationwide system. Parent organization seeks public awareness, engages partners, tries for environmental change in schools; easy implementation.	For the particular site visited, potential impact may be limited due to no sustainability planand low parental support. By addressing these two issues, potential impact would be increased.

Appendix C (Continued).

			AFTERSCHOOL INITIATIVES				
Location	**Physical Activity**	**Nutrition**	**Duration**	**Other**	**Plausibility**	**Feasibility**	**Potential Impact**
Northeast	30 lesson plans for PA; 2x/weekly; lessons last approximately 45-60 minutes sessions to produce MVPA.	Healthy snack component/ partnership with local produce distributor for fresh fruit and vegetables and milk. The grain component of snack varies (e.g., graham crackers, pretzels, chex mix, cookies).	15 weeks; delivered twice yearly—Spring and Fall.	Health literacy section, designed to teach about food and healthy eating, delivered informally and inconsistently. Developmental assets section includes topics of discussion with children; informally delivered	Sound logic for improved physical fitness; links in logic model between activities, outputs and outcomes sound for physical fitness.	Strong administrative support for program implementation	Due to the sound approach in physical activity and fruit intake, the program has potential impact for childhood obesity.
Northeast	40 minutes PA daily (staff expected to participate with children). Games requiring PA.	Nutritious snack daily; nutrition education periodically. Participate in USDA Child Adult Care Feeding Program.	Throughout school year; ongoing year to year.	Parent pledge (eat healthier and engage in PA), staff incentives, game to reinforce healthy snacks being served, staff BMI reduction challenge, family lifestyle food challenge	For children participating daily, it is highly plausible children will receive health benefits because of the required 40 minutes of PA daily.	Parent organization has necessary resources for full implementation; program institutionalized.	Potential impact is high due to the changing of the afterschool environment to promote physical activity and healthy eating.

				($100 groceries, recipes, grocery store trip with RD), family fun nights, newsletters (healthy recipes, games to play).			
Midwest	At least 30 minutes PA daily; 1 flexibility activity, 2 strength activities, 3 cardio activities. CATCH curriculum followed.	At least 1 nutrition lesson or activity per week (e.g., cooking lesson, food pyramid discussion); "healthy snacks and beverages" daily.		"…several features of the planned program that, at the time of the site visit, were not uniformly implemented in all [name] afterschool programs."	Program plausible for obesity because children exposed to 30 minutes PA/day and offering of a healthy snack.	Program has been institutionalized; in need of more CATCH activity kits, space, and equipment to enhance feasibility.	Potential impact could be increased with more training offered to afterschool coordinators who were reported to not have adequate knowledge about nutrition or willingness to participate in PA with the children.
Southeast	PA twice per week.	Nutrition twice per week.		Site visitors observed little nutrition or physical activity intervention taking place.	With more PA and more nutrition activities taking place, the program could produce favorable outcomes.	Feasible program could be implemented as intended, but full implementation not witnessed during site visit.	Potential impact could be increased with more thorough implementation.

Appendix C (Continued).

			AFTERSCHOOL INITIATIVES				
Location	**Physical Activity**	**Nutrition**	**Duration**	**Other**	**Plausibility**	**Feasibility**	**Potential Impact**
Southwest	Daily, 50 to 60 (about 30 minutes in PA) minutes; "physical education standards"; has on staff a retired Physical Education Instructor; Variety of games involving PA.	Nutrition education included in lesson plans.	Throughout school year; ongoing year to year.	70 lesson plans educating children on physical fitness, nutrition, and self-respect.	Program plausible for reducing childhood obesity because of strong PA program component and other events held by parent organization.	Program feasible based on support from multiple school districts, youth groups, non-profits, and local businesses; high level involvement of trained staff.	High potential impact during after school hoursbecause of dedication to PA. Also small potential impact on home environment due to involvement of family during events offered by parent organization.
West	Require 10 minutes of physical activity for every hour of after school programming.	Nutrition standards for snacks served (including vending machines) have been set. Examples include: No more than 35% of calories from fat, no more than 10% from saturated fat No more than 35% sugar by weight No more than 175 calories per serving for	Ongoing.	Annual training to staff and coaches on healthy vending and healthy snacks. Engage community members through youth advocacy and involvement; a community-based advisory group; and Promoturas providing training to parents.	It is highly plausible that this policy can increase accessibility and availability of healthy food options to school-age children. There is some observational data available to support this.	It is feasible to fully implement this intervention as intended in this community. Keys to full implementation include: A political will to support healthy youth. Strong support and participation from community members. Leadership in the partnering organizations.	Potential impact is high. The policies are being implemented in many school-based and non-school-based afterschool programs; there are systems to support and monitor implementation.

		elementary and 250 calories per serving for middle and high schools At least 50% fruit-juice or 50% vegetable-juice based drinks with no added sweetener Water with no added sweetener					
Midwest	60 to 90 minutes each week of physical activity.	60 minutes of nutritional activities and education each week.	Ongoing.	Parental and other adults (e.g., staff) are encouraged to develop a healthy environment; improve self-image and enjoyment of healthy behaviors.	Plausibility is high. Initial evaluation findings show changes in children's physical activity enjoyment, increased health behaviors, and an initial decrease in BMI.	Multiple agencies implement this program. Staff at each agency implement the program, and graduate students collect data and provide technical assistance.	Potential impact is fairly high because of ongoing evaluation efforts. They have modified the program to increase fidelity, sustainability, and collaboration.
Southwest	One hour is dedicated to physical activity each day. The majority is MVPA.	Nutrition education is delivered by a registered dietitian; efforts to serve a healthy snack by collaborating	Program lasts for duration of school year.	Emphasis on cultural awareness; field trips; tobacco prevention; diabetes education.	It is plausible that the program could reduce childhood obesity by ensuring that children spend at least 60 minutes after each school day in MVPA.	Feasibility of implementation is high if there is adequate staff and space to engage in MVPA.	At the time of the site visit, enrollment was limited to 2 schools, but there were plans to increase this. Potential impact is high for participants because of focus on physical activity.

Appendix C (Continued).

			AFTERSCHOOL INITIATIVES				
Location	**Physical Activity**	**Nutrition**	**Duration**	**Other**	**Plausibility**	**Feasibility**	**Potential Impact**
West	Activities typically occur for 30 minutes per day 4 to 5 days/week, and include games from the CATCH and SPARK curricula, other games, or sports such as basketball, volleyball, and soccer.	Nutrition Education (1 hour/week): Activities are included in a nutrition binder that provides materials for each month of the school year. Gardening (1 hour/week): Activities include visits to one of two large gardens owned by the program. Cooking (1 hour/ week): Classes occur at the individual school sites and a kitchen classroom. No Junk Food policy for students and staff (staff who	Program lasts for duration of school year.	Half of the program sites receive 800 to 1,000 pound produce deliveries from a local food bank weekly. Each child takes 3 to 5 pounds home each week.	Plausibility for nutrition improvement is high because nutrition policies and practices appear well-developed. Plausibility for physical activity is unknown because the policies and programs are less well-defined and do not include a requirement for MVPA.	Feasibility of full implementation appears high due to the well-established nature of the communication and training systems. The leaders and administrator meet weekly, and each leader conducts visits to their after school sites.	Potential impact on nutrition is high: the nutrition education, gardening, cooking, junk food policy and produce distribution programs may impact the after school and home environments related to healthy eating.

		violate can be terminated).					
Southwest	There are an estimated 5 to 10 hours of physical activity and/or nutrition education weekly.	Nutrition education.	Program lasts for duration of school year.		Plausibility somewhat limited because the program's primary emphasis is on educating children about the importance and value of good eating and exercise.	Feasibility is varied because of multiple agencies implementing the program. The program offers an important model for delivering an afterschool program via a multi-agency collaboration.	Potential impact could be increased with more emphasis on changing the nutrition and physical activity environments versus emphasizingeducation alone.
DAYCARE INITIATIVES							
Midwest	Participants engage in 20 minutes of vigorous physical activity at least two times per week and 30 minutes of moderate PA daily.	The program provides nutritious options for snacks and nutrition education.	12 weeks.	Parents can participate in the program by working with their children to complete charts of healthy fruit and vegetable choices or by participating in Family Night activities.	It is likely that the program will produce the desired outcomes if they continue to develop and implement an evaluation plan and continue to discuss detailed plans, evaluate goals and progress, and communicate	Feasibility is high because the 12-week nutrition and physical activity curriculum have been packaged into one program book for site leaders. Further, weekly reports of the curriculum items presented to the children	Program impact information has demonstrated increases in the percent of children who engage in moderate and vigorous activity, choose healthy snack options, and improve overall nutrition knowledge.

Appendix C (Continued).

			DAYCARE INITIATIVES				
Location	**Physical Activity**	**Nutrition**	**Duration**	**Other**	**Plausibility**	**Feasibility**	**Potential Impact**
					plans for expansion.	are collected to ensure program fidelity.	
Midwest	Physical activity lessons offered 3 times/week, include three steps: warm-up/auxiliary activity, main event, and cool down/stretching. The main event is intended to provide 20 minutes of continuous activity.	There are six initial 45 minutes nutrition lessons on the following topics: (1) choosing lower calorie alternatives for snacks; (2) choosing one serving of packaged snack food; (3) choosing beverages without added sugar; (4) choosing cereals with a low amount of added sugar; (5) eating fruit; and, (6) eating vegetables and snacking on vegetables.	Program lasts for duration of school year.		The PA strategy can be expected to increase physical activity. The nutrition lessons employ teaching strategies consistent with Social Cognitive Theory. However, plausibility of the nutrition lessons may be limited because education alone tends to have a limited impact on behavior	The program is fully implemented in the area's YMCA program. The program is delivered by 12 dietetic interns, a number which may be too low to reach the 40+ YMCAs offering before and after school care throughout the area.	Potential for impactis high because of the broad reach to all children in the YMCA before and after school programs.

Northeast	Children 12 months+ receive 60 minutes PA daily (children 3 years+ receive 30 minutes structured, total of 60 minutes); SPARK trainings provided to some communities, but not required.	Reduced intake of low nutrient energy dense beverages and fruit juices with intent to reduce caloric intake by 100-200 kcal/day. Children 2 years+ 1% or lower fat milk. 100% fruit juice, 6 ounces. No specific nutrition guidelines, but the health dept will provide the Eat Well Play Hard nutrition program.	Ongoing.	60 minutes limit for TV and screen time. Parents must follow guidelines when bringing food in with children.	Highly plausible the policy will produce favorable outcomes because of the standards set forth and enforcement.	Feasible policy implemented as intended due to support of administrators in ensuring daycare centers are receiving training.	Potential impact is high because of the focus on sugarsweetened beverages, low fat milk, TV time, and PA time.
Northeast	20 to 30 minutes lesson providing opportunity for PA or a new food.	20 to 30 minutes lesson including an interactive presentation by an RD, opportunity for children to try a new food or PA. Follows *Dietary Guidelines for Americans.*	6-10 weeks.	Train child care staff using NAP SACC. Children given a take home sheet that introduces parents to the lesson taught to the child and a recipe.	Program plausible because of multi-components: PA, increased fruit and vegetable and low-fat dairy consumption all stressed.	Program can be implemented with fidelity due to strong organizational support at state and community level as well as strong infrastructure.	Potential impact could be increased with a longer duration and more PA offered to childcare staff to support changes in the social/physical environment of the daycare.

Appendix C (Continued).

			DAYCARE INITIATIVES				
Location	**Physical Activity**	**Nutrition**	**Duration**	**Other**	**Plausibility**	**Feasibility**	**Potential Impact**
Southeast	Brief PA games.	Information on nutrition (both for children and for childcare providers).	Ongoing to various levels of implementa-tion.	Train-the-trainer (county health promotion coordinators and cooperative extension agents trained, who then train child care providers). Trainings offered 1 to 3x/year and last 3 to 4 hours, cost $5	Plausible that children will increase recognition of fruits and vegetables.	Quality packaging of materials, use of trainer's manual, training of childcare providers, provision of free kits to those trained all enhance feasibility of implementation	andwillingness to try new fruits and vegetables. Potential impact for changing the physical or social environment of the daycare is more limited due to limited outreach offered.
West	Children receive PA education and participate in structured PA. Parents and staff receive PA education and may attend classes.	Children, parents, and staff receive nutrition education, recipes, cooking classes, access to community resources; healthier meals, snacks, and beverages served at center; container gardening;	Ongoing.	Health fairs and screening for families and staff; child nutrition assessments: 2 times/year; comprehensive wellness and training activities.	It is plausible that this type of multi-level intervention can produce the desired outcomes. The program hopes to create an environment that supports healthy living.	There is administrative commitment and much energy by staff members. However, fidelity of implementation is unknown due to lack of documentation of key intervention elements.	Potential impact is unknown. During the site visit, limited implementation of unique programming andlittle participation by staff and families was observed.

		targeted and individualized "intervention" among overweight children and those at risk.					
Midwest	Structured physical activity for children to achieve the NASPE goal of 60 minutes per day; a 2-hour training on strategies to improve nutrition and physical activity for children.	A 2-hour training on strategies to improve nutrition and physical activity for children; attempts at menu improvement.	Ongoing.	A toolbox with materials to enhance the program, two technical assistance visits; a parent outreach training; materials to conduct a social marketing campaign .	A pilot study shows this is a plausible program for reaching outcomes for nutrition and physical activity.	The program is being implemented as designed; the designated number of child care centers has been recruited and trainers are delivering the intervention to the child care center staff	Potential impact depends on the trainings and howwell the trainees are implementing the program. Training has beenprovided to approximately 80 centers over the past 2 years.
Southeast	Staff training in curricula to promote healthy eating and physical activity to kids.	Improvement of childcare menus to promote healthy food and beverage options; policies to reduce or eliminate unhealthy options at parties and celebrations.	Ongoing.	Staff wellness initiatives; nutrition and physical activity newsletters are provided to parents on a monthly basis.	It is plausible that the intervention could produce the desired outcomes with rigorous implementation and close monitoring.	It is feasible that the intervention for the childcare centers could be implemented fully as there appears to be buy-in and commitment from childcare center staff	At the time of site visit, full implementation was in progress in3 childcare centers; full implementation could have an impact on eating habits and physical activity.

Appendix C (Continued).

			DAYCARE INITIATIVES				
Location	**Physical Activity**	**Nutrition**	**Duration**	**Other**	**Plausibility**	**Feasibility**	**Potential Impact**
East	A research-to-practice initiative incorporating best practice guidelines such as: NASPE recommendations; Brigh t Futures in Practice-Nutrition and Physical Activity; American Academy of Pediatrics Policy Statements and Task Force on Obesity Strategies; Institute of Medicine Report; & CDC's BMI-for-Age/Gender Screening Guidelines.	See Physical Activity column.	Ongoing.	Training and technical assistance to program staff.	It is plausible that the intervention could lead to healthier eating and physical activity with rigorous implementation and close monitoring.	The training of regional facilitators has the potential to expand the program in an expeditious way.Mechanisms to ensure that the training provided by facilitators is of the same caliber as that provided by the initial core cadre of trainers would ensure quality training is taking place.	At the time of the site visit, 110 facilitators had been trained. There is potential for impact on the social and physical environment to promote active living and healthyeating

References

Barbeau, P., Johnson, M. H., Howe, C. A., Allison, J., Davis, C. L., Gutin, B., et al. (2007). Ten months of exercise improves general and visceral adiposity, bone, and fitness in Black girls. *Obesity*, *15*, 2077- 2085.

California After School Resource Center. (2006). *Physical education model content standards for California public schools, kindergarten through grade twelve.* Sacramento, CA: California Department of Education.

Carver, P. R. & Iruka, I. U. (2006). *After-school programs and activities: 2005 (NCES 2006-076).* Washington, DC: National Center for Education Statistics.

Center for the Childcare Workforce. (2004). *Current data on the salaries and benefits of the U.S. early childhood education workforce.* (Rep. No. Item No. 47-0084). Washington, DC: Author.

Committee on Nutrition Standards for Foods in Schools Food and Nutrition Board. (2007). *Nutrition standards for foods in schools: Leading the way toward healthier youth.* Washington, DC: The National Academies Press.

Committee on Prevention of Obesity in Children and Youth. (2005). *Preventing childood obesity: Health in the balance.* Washington, DC: The National Academies Press.

Committee on Sports Medicine and Fitness and Committee on School Health. (2001). Organized sports for children and preadolescents. *Pediatrics*, *107*, 1459-1462.

Freedman, D. S., Dietz, W. H., Srinivasan, S. & Berenson, G. S. (1999). The relation of overweight to cardiovascular risk factors among children and adolescents: The Bogalusa Heart Study. *Pediatrics*, *103*, 1175-1182.

Fuller, C., Keller, L., Olson, J. & Plymale, A. (2005). Helping preschoolers become healthy eaters. *Journal of Pediatric Health Care*, *19*, 178-182.

Kelder, S., Hoelscher, D. M., Barroso, C. S., Walker, J. L., Cribb, P. & Hu, S. (2005). The CATCH Kids Club: A pilot after-school study for improving elementary students' nutrition and physical activity. *Public Health Nutrition*, *8*, 133-140.

McKenzie, T. L., Feldman, H. A., Woods, S. E., Romero, K. A., Dahlstrom, V., Stone, E. J., et al. (1995). Children's activity levels and lesson context during third-grade physical education. *Research Quarterly for Exercise and Sport*, *66*, 184-193.

Nader, P. R. (2003). Frequency and intensity of activity of third-grade children in physical education. *Archives of Pediatrics & Adolescent Medicine*, *157*, 185-190.

National Association for Sport and Physical Education. (2002). *Active start: A statement of physical activity guidelines for children birth to five years.* Reston, VA: Author.

National Association for Sport and Physical Education. (2004). *Physical activity for children: A statement of guidelines for children ages 5-12.* (2nd ed.) Reston, VA: Author.

National Association of Child Care Resource & Referral Agencies. (2008). Child care in America: 2008 State fact sheets. Arlington, VA: Author.

Ogden, C. L., Carroll, M. D. & Flegal, K. M. (2008). High body mass index for age among US children and adolescents, 2003-2006. *Journal of the American Medical Association, 299,* 240 1-2405.

Pate, R. R., Pfeiffer, K. A., Trost, S., Ziegler, P. & Dowda, M. (2004). Physical activity among children attending preschools. *Pediatrics, 114,* 1258-1263.

Patrick, K., Spear, B., Holt, K. & Sofka, D. (2001). *Bright futures in practice: Physical activity.* Arlington, VA: National Center for Education in Maternal and Child Health.

Patton, M. (1997). *Utilization-focused evaluation: The new century text.* Thousand Oaks: Sage Publications.

Scientific Software Development GmbH. (2008). ATLAS.ti Scientific Software Development GmbH [Computer software]. Berlin, Germany: Author.

Story, M., Holt, K. & Sofka, D. (2002). *Bright futures in practice: Nutrition* (2nd ed.). Arlington, VA: National Center for Education in Maternal and Child Health.

Story, M., Kaphingst, K. M. & French, S. (2006). The role of child care settings in obesity prevention. *Future Child, 16,* 143-168.

Tides Center. (2009). CANFIT: Nutrition. Retrieved from http://canfit.org/our_work/nutrition

U.S. Department of Agriculture. (2008). Child & adult care food program. Retrieved from http://www.fns.usda.gov/cnd/Care/CACFP/aboutcacfp.htm

U.S. Department of Health and Human Services. (2000). *Healthy People 2010: Understanding and improving health.* (2nd ed). Washington, DC: U.S. Government Printing Office.

U.S. Department of Health and Human Services. (2008a). *2008 Physical activity guidelines for Americans.* Washington, DC: U.S. Department of Health and Human Services.

U.S. Department of Health and Human Services. (2008b). Physical activity guidelines for Americans: Federal Resources—Children and Adolescents. Retrieved from http://www.health federalresources.aspx#Children

U.S. Department of Health and Human Services & U.S. Department of Agriculture. (2005). *Dietary guidelines for Americans* (Rep. No. 6th ed.). Washington, DC: U.S. Government Printing Office.

Welk, G. J. & Meredith, M. D. (2008). *Fitnessgram/Activitygram reference guide* (3rd ed.). Dallas, TX: The Cooper Institute.

Wholey, J. S. (2004). Evaluability assessment. In J. S., Wholey, H. P. Hatry, & K. E.. Newcomer, (Eds.), *Handbook of practical program evaluation*, (33-62). San Francisco: Jossey-Bass.

Yin, Z., Hanes, J., Jr., Moore, J. B., Humbles, P., Barbeau, P. & Gutin, B. (2005a). An after-school physical activity program for obesity prevention in children: The Medical College of Georgia FitKid Project. *Evaluation & the Health Professions*, *28*, 67-89.

Yin, Z., Gutin, B., Johnson, M. H., Hanes, J., Moore, J. B., Cavnar, M., et al. (2005b). An environmental approach to obesity prevention in children: Medical College of Georgia FitKid Project year 1 results. *Obesity Research*, *13*, 2153-2161.

In: Prevention of Childhood Obesity
Editor: Christina V. Mancuso, pp. 43-99
ISBN: 978-1-61209-962-0

Chapter 2

ACCESS TO HEALTHY FOODS

Christina V. Mancuso

ACKNOWLEDGMENTS

Early Assessment of Programs and Policies to Prevent Childhood Obesity is a collaboration of the Robert Wood Johnson Foundation (RWJF); the Centers for Disease Control and Prevention's (CDC) Division of Nutrition, Physical Activity and Obesity (DNPAO), Division of Adolescent and School Health (DASH), and Division of Adult and Community Health (DACH) Prevention Research Centers (PRC) Program Office; and the CDC Foundation. ICF Macro, an ICF International Company, serves as the coordinating center for the project. The team receives guidance from a Funder's Advisory Committee, which includes representatives from the U.S. Department of Agriculture (USDA), National Institutes of Health's (NIH's) National Cancer Institute (NCI), the Kellogg Foundation, Kaiser Permanente, and members of CDC and RWJF not otherwise involved in the project.

This report was made possible by the participation of program staff and others who welcomed members of our project team to their sites, answered our questions, and allowed us to observe their programs. We are grateful to the staff in the field who overcome the daily challenges of program implementation. Theodore Roosevelt eloquently said, "It is not the critic who counts. ... The credit belongs to the man who is actually in the arena, whose face is marred by dust and sweat and blood, who strives valiantly, who errs and comes up short again and again, because there is no effort without error or shortcoming, but who knows the great enthusiasms, the great devotions, who spends himself for a worthy cause." Much energy and enthusiasm is devoted to this exemplary work. We are grateful to the program staff members and applaud their tremendous efforts put forth in increasing access to healthier foods in underserved areas.

I. INTRODUCTION

The Early Assessment of Programs and Policies to Prevent Childhood Obesity was a 2-year project to identify and assess local-level programs and policies to prevent obesity that have been implemented with notable success. We focused on promising environmental interventions implemented in community settings intended to improve the eating habits and physical activity levels of children aged 3 to 17 years. We gave priority to programs that addressed low-income populations and ethnic groups that experience disproportionate childhood obesity.

Purpose of the Systematic Screening and Assessment Method

The evidence base for environmental interventions is very limited, and communities and schools are implementing a wide variety of interventions with little guidance about effective practices. Scans performed by the National Council of State Legislatures; the Kellogg and Dell Foundations; State health departments; and schools as well as activities funded by CDC, NIH, and USDA reveal that hundreds of environmental interventions are being implemented across the country. While those scans are extremely useful for providing a broad picture of trends and interventions, they do not uncover the most exemplary or innovative environmental interventions. The Systematic Screening and Assessment (SSA) Method is a new evaluation approach to identify and assess several innovations being implemented in the field within a relatively short period of time. Innovations are assessed both for their potential impact on health outcomes and their readiness for evaluation.

As part of the SSA Method, evaluability assessments were used to assess the plausibility and feasibility of selected programs and policies that were identified as promising during the search process and selected by the project's expert panel. Evaluability assessment (EA) is a process in which evaluators work with program administrators and stakeholders to help them to prepare for evaluation (Patton, 1997). The process clarifies goals, clarifies program design by specifying the program model, determines stakeholders' views on the important issues, and explores program reality (Wholey, 2004). EAs can help to determine whether a rigorous evaluation study is feasible and merited for a particular program or policy. As such, they can help to avoid premature investment in rigorous evaluation of programs or policies that have not been adequately implemented and allow evaluation resources to be targeted to programs or policies deemed ready for rigorous evaluation.

Focus Areas

The Funder's Advisory Committee identified three thematic areas of interest during the first year of the project: (1) child care programs and policies in afterschool and day care settings, (2) programs or policies that increase access to healthier foods, and (3) school district local wellness policies. During the second year, project staff identified two additional topic areas: (1) comprehensive school physical activity and (2) the built environment.

This synthesis report focuses on programs that were designed to increase access to affordable, higher-quality, less-calorie-dense foods in low-income communities during the 2 years of the project. The programs were groundbreaking because they strived to improve health in venues typically driven by sales and profit. Our criteria and winnowing process identified promising programs for increasing access to healthier foods in lower-income communities. Those programs fostered collaboration to improve the health of their communities and, as one component of a more comprehensive approach, have potential to enhance nutrition for children aged 3 to 17 years. In this report, we synthesize findings from EAs of 16 programs; provide insights for further program development and evaluation; and describe environmental interventions in farmers markets, restaurants, and supermarkets or convenience stores. While our findings may not apply to every project that aims to make healthy food accessible, some common themes emerged from this work.

II. The Problem: Obesity and Access to Healthy Foods

According to data from the National Health and Nutrition Examination Survey (NHANES), which is designed to assess the health and nutritional status of adults and children in the United States through interviews and physical examinations, our nation is experiencing a rise in childhood obesity. Data from NHANES (1976 to 1980 and 2003 to 2006) suggested that the prevalence of obesity has more than doubled for children aged 2 to 5 years, from 5.0% to 12.4%. For those aged 6 to 11 years, the prevalence of obesity increased from 6.5% to 17.0%; and for those aged 12 to 19 years, the prevalence increased from 5.0% to 17.6% (Ogden, Carroll, & Flegal, 2008; Centers for Disease Control and Prevention, 2006). Further, obesity-associated annual hospital costs for children and youth have more than tripled over two decades, rising from $35 million in 1979 to 1981 to $127 million in 1997 to 1999. The Institute of Medicine (2004) declared that prevention of obesity in children and youths should be a national public health priority.

The number of calories people consume in the United States has increased in the past 30 years, and the rise is likely related to people eating more unhealthy foods (Cutler, Glaeser, & Shapiro, 2003). Many adults and children have unhealthy diets, particularly those living in low-income urban neighborhoods where supermarkets and affordable quality produce are scarce (Powell, Slater, Mirtcheva, Bao, & Chaloupka, 2007). Researchers have shown that low-income communities offer limited access to supermarkets and fresh produce and greater access to convenience or liquor stores, as compared with wealthier neighborhoods (Moore & Diez Roux, 2006). Research also suggests that people living in neighborhoods with better access to supermarkets and limited access to convenience stores tend to have healthier diets and lower levels of obesity (Larson, Story, & Nelson, 2008). Families who have easy access to affordable, high-quality fruits and vegetables are more likely to consume them (Sallis & Glanz, 2006). In contrast, families and children from lower socioeconomic backgrounds are less likely to have diets that meet nutrition guidelines for good health and are at higher risk for obesity (Darmon & Drewnowski, 2008; Turrell, Hewitt, Patterson, & Oldenburg, 2003; Ogden et al., 2006; Miech et al., 2006; Wang & Beydoun, 2007). In addition, these populations often suffer disproportionately from diet-related diseases such as type 2 diabetes, hypertension, and coronary heart disease; one factor that may contribute to this finding is the lack of access to healthy foods (Swinburn, Metcalf, & Ley, 2001; Taubes, 1997).

In many communities, healthy foods and fresh produce are not as widely available as fast food and other foods high in calories but low in nutrition (Lewis et al., 2005; Horowitz, Colson, Hebert, & Lancaster, 2004; Morland, Wing, & Diez Roux, 2002). Fast-food chains, corner stores, or bodegas are often the only sources of food in communities with high rates of poverty. Low-income neighborhoods have only one-half to one-third as many supermarkets as higher-wealth areas; and neighborhoods that are predominantly African American or Latino are less likely to have supermarkets than White neighborhoods (Morland, Wing, Diez Roux, & Poole, 2002). In addition, the size, physical condition, and nutritional content of merchandise in the stores of low-income neighborhoods tend to be poorer than that of wealthier neighborhoods (Kolodinsky & Cranwell, 2000). Healthy foods such as whole grains, low-fat dairy products, and fresh fruits and vegetables may be less available and more expensive in poor minority neighborhoods than in wealthy White neighborhoods (Moore & Diez Roux, 2006). The lack of access to affordable and healthy foods may be contributing to disparities in diet-related chronic diseases and obesity rates.

Good nutrition is a vital component of health, well-being, and quality of life. However, in 2002, more than 35 million Americans experienced limited access to nutritious food on a regular basis (Institute of Medicine, 2004). There is a clear link between diet and the availability of affordable, nutritious food; a number of studies have found that neighborhood residents who have better access to supermarkets tend to have healthier diets (Bodor, Rose, Farley, Swalm, & Scott, 2008; Morland, Wing, & Diez Roux, 2002; Wang, Kim, Gonzalez, MacLeod, & Winkleby, 2007). Supermarkets often offer the greatest variety of healthy, high-quality products at the lowest cost, and shoppers generally prefer supermarkets to smaller grocery stores and convenience stores (Food Marketing Institute, 2006; Bodor et al., 2008). Researchers have found that for each additional supermarket in a neighborhood, African Americans' fruit and vegetable consumption increased by 32% (Morland, Wing, & Diez Roux, 2002). The health of children and families is affected when their neighborhood does not have a grocery store with fresh fruits and vegetables available (Mikkelsen & Chehimi, 2007). The main reasons for the lack of access to affordable and healthy foods in low-income neighborhoods are the relocation of full-service supermarkets to suburbs, lack of transportation, and a proliferation of convenience stores offering a limited selection of healthy foods at higher prices (Koplan, Liverman, & Kraak, 2005).

Farmers markets are becoming more common and are one avenue to providing fresh, locally grown produce to many communities. Between 1994 and

2008, the number of farmers markets increased 167%, from 1,755 to 4,685 (U.S. Department of Agriculture, 2007). The USDA's Farmers Market Nutrition Program (FMNP) seeks to provide fresh, nutritious, locally grown fruits and vegetables to Women, Infant, and Children (WIC) participants and senior citizens, and to expand the awareness and use of farmers markets. In addition to their regular WIC benefits, under FMNP, participants and senior citizens receive $10 to $30 per year to spend on produce at farmers markets; States may provide additional financial support. The financial assistance allows families to purchase fresh fruits and vegetables that they might not be able to afford otherwise. In an attempt to better serve the needs of poor communities, local farmers markets have also started to accept electronic benefit transfer (EBT, or food stamps) in addition to WIC and senior-citizen farmers market coupons. Currently, 46 States have at least one farmers market accepting EBT transactions (U.S. Department of Agriculture, 2007). According to USDA, the number of farmers markets across the country accepting EBT transactions increased from 532 in 2007 to 605 as of June 2008.

In addition to the lack of access to fresh and affordable healthful foods, many low-income neighborhoods have an abundant supply of fast-food restaurants. Poorer neighborhoods with a higher percentage of African American residents have more fast-food restaurants than their wealthier counterparts (Lewis et al., 2005), and these restaurants typically have few healthy options (foods high in nutritional quality and low in calories) available (Block, Scribner, & DeSalvo, 2004). In general, foods prepared away from home tend to be more calorie dense and of poorer nutritional quality (Guthrie, Lin, & Frazao, 2002). Adults and children consume more calories, more fat, more fried foods, more soft drinks, fewer fruits and vegetables, and less fiber when eating restaurant foods than when eating meals prepared at home (Schwartz & Brownell, 2007). Various studies have linked frequent eating out to higher caloric intake, weight gain, and obesity (Bowman, Gortmaker, Ebbeling, Pereira, & Ludwig, 2004; MacCrory, Fuss, Hays, Vinken, Greenberg, & Roberts, 1999; Pereira et al., 2005). Several studies also have shown that fast-food restaurants tend to cluster in school neighborhoods; 68% of the 1,718 schools in the 20 largest U.S. cities are within walking distance of at least one fast-food restaurant (Larson, Story, & Nelson, 2008). One way to mitigate these issues is for full-service and fast-food restaurants to provide or expand healthier—and appetizing—food options. Increasing the availability and identification of healthy foods on restaurant menus is one strategy to encourage consumers to make healthy choices in restaurants. However, as businesses, restaurants identify their most important priorities as expanding sales and increasing profits, so they will only offer healthy food options if there is adequate consumer demand (Glanz, Sallis, Saelens, & Frank, 2007).

Despite such findings, the evaluation of food away from home and fast-food dining in relation to obesity among children is limited. While some authors have shown a relationship between frequency of consumption of food from fast-food restaurants in girls aged 8 to 19 years and the development of obesity (Thomson et al., 2004), more studies are needed to establish the evidence base of the food environment and dietary factors related to childhood obesity (Newby, 2007). Although several models exist for changing environments and policies in restaurants to increase nutritious eating behaviors, most have not been systematically evaluated. More studies are needed to establish what types of restaurant interventions can be used to prevent obesity among children.

Some cities are attempting to improve their community food environments by offering grants, loans, and tax benefits to stimulate the development of neighborhood groceries in underserved urban neighborhoods; initiating farmers markets; and making healthier products available in restaurants and stores. Improved access to and affordability of fruits and vegetables for low-income populations, and increased availability and affordability of healthful foods and beverages at supermarkets, grocery stores, restaurants, and farmers markets are two intermediate goals toward reducing obesity through policy and environmental changes.

Little research on food access has explicitly examined obesity as an outcome although there is a strong relationship between obesity prevention and a healthy diet (i.e., the consumption of fruit and vegetables and limited fat intake). For many environmental, policy, and societal variables, carefully designed evaluations of ongoing programs and policies will help to answer key questions about the intended effects of obesity interventions. The challenge is to identify which interventions, programs, and policies are promising and have the greatest potential impact in efforts to curb the obesity epidemic. Through EAs, the project team sought to provide better understanding of the current interventions, programs, and policies targeted at increasing access to healthy foods.

III. Methods

Nomination and Selection of Programs/Policies

In spring 2007, the Early Assessment project team solicited nominations of environmental programs and policies aimed at increasing access to healthier foods in low-income communities. After a comprehensive scan to identify promising practices, we issued a call for nominations to public health professionals and researchers, supplemented by inventories of environmental interventions maintained by CDC, RWJF, and other organizations. Programs and policies were selected for further review if they met the following inclusion criteria: (a) were environmental interventions, (b) were implemented by late 2007; (c) had not already undergone rigorous evaluation, and (d) were not strict replications of a promising or evidence-based model. The staff compiled brief descriptions of interventions that met the inclusion criteria for review by an expert panel.

In June 2007, the project team convened a panel of 15 experts in evaluation, measurement, nutrition, physical activity, school-aged youths, and community programs. The expert panel used the following criteria to rate and select programs and policies for an EA:

- Assessment
- Potential impact
- Innovation
- Reach to target population
- Acceptability to stakeholders
- Feasibility of implementation
- Feasibility of adoption
- Intervention sustainability
- Generalizability
- Staff/organizational capacity

Those criteria are further described in Appendix A. During the first year of the project, a total of 55 food access programs were nominated; 22 met the criteria for inclusion, and 10 were selected to participate in an EA. Of the 10 programs selected, 1 did not participate because of a staffing change.

The nomination and selection process was repeated during the second year of the project. In 2008, the project team received 13 nominations for food access programs, and 9 met the criteria for inclusion. The expert panel recommended all

9 programs for an EA. Of the 9 programs selected, 2 did not participate because of a delayed start in program implementation or other logistical issues. In total, the team conducted EAs of 16 food access programs.

Evaluability Assessment Site Visits

Each EA involved (1) a review of background documentation about the program or policy; (2) the development of a program or policy logic model to outline program goals and activities; and (3) a 2.5-day site visit, in which trained site visitors assessed implementation, data collection, and evaluation capacity through interviews with program staff and partners. In general, interviewees discussed the program goals, current activities, data collection efforts, staffing, funding, challenges, and successes. The project team and expert panel reviewed the findings from all the EAs to determine the degree of promise of the various programs and policies and their readiness for rigorous evaluation.

Logic Model

As part of the EA, site visitors developed logic models to visually represent the logic or theory of a program or policy. The logic models linked program resources and activities to expected outcomes and goals. If programs already had their own logic models, site visitors used these models as a basis to discuss progress of implementation. For programs that did not have an existing logic model, site visitors developed a draft logic model based on document review before the visit. Site visitors used the logic models to clarify their understanding of program components and to elicit feedback from program staff. The EA team revised the logic models as they learned more about the program through interviews and observations during the site visit.

Site visitors spent the last day of their visit debriefing with relevant stakeholders on preliminary findings from the interviews and reviewing the logic model. Often, key stakeholders such as program leadership (e.g., director and coordinator), program staff (e.g., nutritionists, educators, and evaluator), and community partners participated in these discussions. After each discussion about program activities, outcomes, goals, and evaluation capacity, site visitors and program staff revised the logic model to ensure it accurately reflected the program. For example, during one debriefing session, site visitors met with the program staff to review the logic model and to discuss how program activities would lead to intended outcomes. In this collaborative and interactive process, site visitors used colored index cards to represent each category of the logic model (inputs, activities, etc.) and worked with program staff to expand on or clarify all components of the logic model. Together, program staff and the EA team went through the logic model to ensure that each input had an associated activity or process, outputs, and outcomes. The team added processes as a category of inputs, to reflect the fact that many of the activities were ongoing iterative processes rather than single endeavors. As they physically constructed the logic model on a large table, moving and rewriting cards, both program staff and the site visitors found that on several occasions, they had to go back to add an input or activity to match a later output or outcome. This iterative process captured the most relevant aspects of the initiative in the logic model.

Data Sources and Analysis

Primary data sources for this synthesis report were program nominations, expert panel preliminary reviews and perspectives, reports written by site visitors, logic models, and expert panel postsite reviews and recommendations. Reports were analyzed for themes using open coding (Bernard, 2000). Three team members were involved in the initial identification of codes. Each individual developed codes independently after reviewing two sets of reports, then compared and discussed similarities and differences to arrive at a single comprehensive list of codes for analysis (Patton, 2002). One team member then coded all reports for each thematic area. ATLAS.ti (version 5.0) was used to categorize and sort data within codes. Site visitors reviewed a draft of the common themes and provided feedback to help refine or add to the findings.

IV. Results

Context of Programs

During the 2 years of the project, the team conducted EAs of 5 supermarket programs, 1 corner store program, 5 farmers markets, and 5 restaurant programs. State or local health departments developed and implemented 8 of the 16 programs that were examined. The remaining programs were developed and implemented by nonprofit and private organizations whose missions include promoting healthy communities, promoting healthy eating, and providing health care to underserved populations. One program was developed by a retail supermarket chain.

While programs varied in their activities, all had a common goal of increasing access or awareness of healthier food items. To provide context, each program is briefly described below.

Supermarkets and Corner Stores

- One supermarket initiative provided financing or distribution mechanisms to help establish or renovate supermarkets in low-income areas.
- A resident-led, community-based development organization transformed distressed communities and neighborhoods and helped to place a full-size chain supermarket in the area.
- One supermarket was a locally owned and operated full-service cooperative grocery store with a nutrition education center.
- A regional chain of supermarkets developed a navigation system to rate food items based on nutrient density to help consumers make more informed decisions
- One initiative was a neighborhood watch program in which community members worked with the food retailer manager to promote healthy foods and rate grocery stores' selection of health foods.
- The corner store program increased availability of healthier items, such as 1% milk and fruits and vegetables, by helping owners change their inventory.

Farmers Markets

- Three farmers market programs sought to increase access to fresh fruits and vegetables with the acceptance of food assistance benefits.
- One farmers market offered an incentive program to encourage the purchase of fruits and vegetables at farmers markets, and one had a direct-to-consumer produce distribution system.

Restaurants

- One restaurant initiative was a citywide regulation requiring food service establishments with more than 15 locations nationally to post the calorie content of their menu items.
- The remaining four restaurant programs provided or highlighted healthier menu options for consumers.

Target Audience

Thirteen of the 16 programs targeted—or were located in—predominantly low-income areas with large minority populations. While the remaining three programs (two restaurant and one supermarket program) did not directly focus on socioeconomically or racially disparate populations, program staff believed that their efforts could help to alleviate the disparities in the prevalence of overweight and obesity. Although those programs did not directly target children, they affect children's health because parents and family members who are the programs' target audience purchase most of the food children eat and often reinforce and support healthy or unhealthy eating (Golan & Crow, 2004; Golan, Weizman, Apter, & Fainaru, 1998). The staff in all 16 programs referenced consumers as the primary beneficiary or stakeholder of their intervention. In addition, the staff of some programs mentioned community leaders, health professionals, restaurant and store owners, and the local government as other groups with a stake in the program.

Reach

Many of the programs had few data about the reach to the target population. Therefore, it was not clear what proportion of households in a given low-income neighborhood was shopping in the supermarkets/corner stores, using farmers markets, or patronizing restaurants. However, many site visitors felt that reach was low for the programs they visited. One site visitor commented, "The program currently reaches a small percent of the low-income target audience. The population of the city is expansive, and the program is not yet at the scale [where it can] make a significant entrée into this population."

On the other hand, two restaurant initiatives and one supermarket program appeared to have extensive reach as well as the potential to expand their reach. The initiative requiring restaurants with more than 15 locations nationally to post the calorie content on their menu items is a citywide policy, affecting about 3,000 of the city's 23,000 food service establishments. Prior studies from the city's health department have indicated that the 3,000 food service establishments required to post calorie information serve about 35% of purchased meals. Therefore, program staff expect the initiative to reach a significant portion of restaurant consumers. Site visitors noted that if implemented in other settings, a similar regulation is likely to also have broad reach, varying in relation to the proportion of residents who purchase meals from restaurants. Another restaurant initiative has partnered with a local McDonald's to highlight the healthier options on its menu. If the initiative is adopted by other McDonald's franchises, the program has the potential for national reach. Lastly, the supermarket that developed a food rating system hopes to license and offer it to other supermarkets across the country. The potential reach is high if supermarkets across the country (including big chain supermarkets) adopt the system. Further, if the program provokes food manufacturers to reformulate their items so they meet the nutrient-rich rating criteria, then the potential reach is very high.

Logic Model of Access to Healthy Food Initiatives

Program and policy administrators, stakeholders, and staff worked with the site visitors to develop a logic model of their initiative. Staff at four programs had already developed their own logic models before the EAs and shared them with site visitors. As necessary, site visitors and program staff refined or developed a site's logic model to accurately describe the program or policy. Appendix B provides an example logic model for the access to health food initiatives. This section describes three components of the logic model: (1) goals and anticipated outcomes, (2) inputs, and (3) activities.

Goals and Anticipated Outcomes

In general, childhood obesity prevention was cited as priority for many programs and their communities. Programs had different settings and scopes, but all shared the goal of providing healthier food or increasing awareness of healthier food choices by making the foods more physically accessible and more affordable. In one program, staff explained that the overall goal of their activities was to "make the healthy choice the easy choice." Another program was described as a "yellow brick road" to help consumers navigate through the confusion of nutrition-related messages in the media, in advertisements, and on food packaging and guide them to healthy food choices. While all 16 programs aimed to increase access to or raise awareness of healthier foods, 7 also explicitly aimed to improve health outcomes by reducing obesity and diet-related diseases such as diabetes and heart disease.

Three supermarket initiatives also sought to stimulate economic development and increase social capital of their communities. Through their work in developing supermarkets in underserved communities, the three programs hope to create jobs for local residents, revitalize commercial real estate, leverage private sector capital, and increase property values in the area. The supermarkets will also provide lower-cost, nutritional foods and savings on transportation for neighborhood residents. In addition to contributing to a system of greater food security and economic empowerment in the community, one of the supermarket programs stated that it also aims to improve the financial sustainability of local farmers.

Another program sought to be the premier nutrition navigation system for the nation, contributing to improving the health and wellness of consumers. Because the supermarket had invested time, money, and effort into developing a nutrition rating system, it is reasonable that another program goal was to increase profits and sales. Because many of the food access programs were implemented in business venues typically driven by profit, the supermarket held a unique view of health as a priority.

With all 16 programs, there was unanimous agreement among program staff on the logic models developed during the evaluability assessment. The high level of agreement among program staff and partners on program goals was noteworthy and demonstrated that stakeholders had a shared understanding about what the program was attempting to do. The clarity and agreement about goals was a strength of all the programs.

Inputs

Funding

Funding varied greatly among the sites visited, and specific amounts were not provided for all programs. From the available information, funding amounts ranged from tens of thousands of dollars for four of the restaurant programs to millions of dollars for four of the supermarket initiatives. Regarding one farmers market program, site visitors noted, "The program seems to run efficiently on a lean budget and staffing and would need more resources to undertake [its] challenges." Many program staff felt that their funding was insufficient for carrying out activities beyond planning and implementation. Almost half of the programs lacked funds for any type of evaluation activities.

Major sources of funding for these programs included grants from the government (USDA, Housing and Urban Development [HUD], CDC, State or local health departments), community- based organizations, private organizations, and foundations (WK Kellogg, Kaiser Permanente, Komen, William Penn, Walter and Elise Haas). Other sources included grants from universities, individual donors, and banks. The supermarket item rating system received all its funding in-house from the parent company, a food retailer. Financial support for farmers markets appeared to be the most limited, with the USDA Food Stamp Nutrition Education Program as the primary source of funding. All programs would benefit from increased funding to expand or augment program planning, implementation, and evaluation activities.

Site visitors felt that five of the programs were sustainable, in part because they appeared to have a sound business plan and would not rely on outside funding after initial startup. For the remaining programs, sustainability would likely depend on continued funding, documentation of positive community impact, and continued engagement and support from the community. For one restaurant program, site visitors felt that the sustainability of the program depended on the current program director. The program relied heavily on her as a champion. The future of the program could be in doubt if the program director were to leave and not be replaced by someone who shared her passion for the program and had the skill set necessary to keep the program operational.

Staffing and Resources

Programs staffed between one and five full-time equivalents. Some programs, particularly restaurants and farmers markets, relied heavily on volunteers to assist with outreach and marketing activities. The leadership and staff of one restaurant program described their efforts as resource- intensive. It required significant travel and recruitment efforts outside the office and during nontraditional work hours. Site visitors noted that it was necessary to have a sound, well-rooted organization as the flagship for the program. Whether it was the State or local health department, or a private nonprofit organization, it was important that the parent organization had a strong presence in the community. All programs were situated within mature, respected parent organizations that sought to provide strong support in terms of administrative and content expertise. Staff members were very dedicated to their programs. However, stakeholders of many programs indicated that having more staff and funding available would better facilitate full implementation of their programs.

All sites were receptive and interested in evaluation, although few had appropriated funds to conduct a process or outcome evaluation. If funding were provided, however, site visitors reported that 10 of the 16 programs would have the capacity to participate in and support a rigorous evaluation. Those 10 programs had knowledgeable staff with the skills and interest to participate in a comprehensive evaluation. Most programs were housed within reputable organizations with evaluation experience.

Partnerships

All programs—supermarkets, corner stores, farmers markets, and restaurants—had constructive and beneficial relationships with various partners, including universities and colleges, local and State departments of health, local governments, advocacy groups, trade associations, community-based organizations, neighborhood associations, private businesses, and wholesale food distributors and vendors. All programs reported a high degree of support from their partners as well as the community. During interviews with site visitors, partners were positive about their collaborative relationships with the parent organizations in planning and implementing the interventions, and they understood the value of that work. Farmers and vendors, restaurant owners, and supermarket operators and store owners were willing to engage and participate in interventions aimed at preventing obesity and its related chronic conditions. On the basis of self-reports from a few program staff, it appeared that many consumers also understood the benefits of increased access to healthier foods.

The neighborhood watch program relied on community members to rate grocery stores' selection of foods and to work with stores to promote healthy foods. It required an intense effort from community members, many of whom appeared to be very supportive of the program. The program developed partnerships with community-based organizations including churches, youth-focused groups, community development groups, advocacy groups, universities, and health care groups. Likewise, program staff of the supermarket food rating system partnered with many community organizations—afterschool programs, medical providers, and the local department of health—which helped to provide credibility to the rating system.

Though it had collaborative relationships with a variety of partners, the calorie labeling initative also had some opponents. The local restaurant association filed a lawsuit in a U.S. District Court claiming that the new ordinance was preempted by Federal law and, more broadly, that it violated the First Amendment. The District Court overturned the measure in September 2007, ruling that Federal law did preempt it as written. In October 2007 the health department submitted a second calorie-posting proposal. The new measure still required that certain restaurants post calorie information on menus and menu boards, but it was written to provide the specific mandatory components that would avoid overlap with the existing FDA regulation. The local restaurant association again sued in February 2008, asking the U.S. District Court to overturn the revised calorie-posting measure. The judge ruled in favor of the regulation in April 2008. While it had initially experienced resistance from the restaurant community, the initiative had also received thousands of written comments in favor of its enactment. Notably, leading national and local professional societies, academic institutions, local hospitals, and advocacy groups applauded the passage of the regulation.

Activities

With one exception, it appeared that all programs were fully implemented or on track for full implementation as proposed by the original program design. Four programs had been pilot tested, and changes to promotional materials, outreach efforts, and data collection were made accordingly as staff better understood how their efforts could be made easier or more effective. About half of the programs expected to expand their efforts by enlarging current sites or implementing the program in new sites. Some programs evolved as they faced challenges with implementation, but the core concepts and goals remained the same. Overall, programs aimed to increase access, awareness, and purchases of healthy food. Other expected outcomes included improved, positive attitudes toward healthy eating; increased consumption of fruits and vegetables; and increased sales of healthy items in supermarkets, corner stores, farmers markets, and restaurants. More detailed information about the activities, outputs, and outcomes of different types of programs follows. Descriptions of the programs are also available in Appendix C.

Supermarkets and Corner Stores

As mentioned previously, we conducted EAs of five supermarket and one corner store program. Three programs were similar initiatives that worked to build or renovate supermarkets in underserved neighborhoods. The other programs were a navigation system developed by a supermarket chain to rate food items based on nutrient density and a neighborhood watch program in which community members worked with the food retailer manager to promote healthy foods and rate grocery stores' selection of health foods. The corner store program increased the inventory of skim milk and fruits and vegetables.

By helping businesses in low-income settings to obtain loan rates and terms that were more flexible and generous than those of commercial lenders, one initiative helped to meet the financing needs of supermarket operators who plan to operate in underserved communities where infrastructure costs and credit needs cannot be fulfilled by conventional financial institutions alone. Staff members of this innovative supermarket initiative received applications for grants or loans from local store operators. Program staff worked directly with the supermarket industry, developers, and underserved communities to match the appropriate projects to each area and lend support throughout the process. Staff members also conducted community outreach to obtain buy-in and establish task forces for the neighborhood to take ownership of the effort. However, many of the neighborhoods where stores were established had low workforce capacity. Store operators often found it difficult to provide sufficient job training (for example, in customer service) for individuals who had never held a job before. Currently, program staff members work with a community- building nonprofit organization to help provide technical assistance and workforce development to store operators. This local organization has been instrumental in helping prepare and place disadvantaged men, women, and teens in appropriate jobs in the supermarkets, with a focus on job retention. In addition, some stores have been models of operator responsiveness to community needs—for example, they provide bundled health and social services, including enrollment in public assistance programs, health insurance outreach, and tax preparation.

Another initiative sought to develop and operate a cooperative food market, train worker-owners for the store, provide nutrition education to customers and the community, purchase and sell produce from local marginalized farmers, maintain a cooperative economic investment program, and market the store to and engage local residents. The market was intended to be a locally owned, community-driven, cooperative grocery store that offered healthy, affordable food and nutrition education. The project leadership believed that local ownership should be a cornerstone of redevelopment efforts. Rather than bringing in national chain supermarkets and convenience stores, they believed that if redevelopment projects are locally owned, they can be used to empower the community, increase work and business skills, and promote economic self-sufficiency for individual residents and the community. With the cooperative model, the business was jointly owned and operated, and profits were shared by members of the cooperative. In addition, the market also planned to offer a cooperative economic investment program, an individual development account (IDA) to provide multilevel investment for community residents. In general, IDAs are matched savings accounts that enable low-income individuals and families to save, build assets, and enter the financial mainstream. This mechanism allowed the worker-owners and community residents to use the store to build financial assets and also fostered community ownership of the market. Under this financial arrangement, one-third of the profits per year from the market will be put into a special bank investment account from which community residents, including worker-owners, can apply to draw a specified proportion of the funds that they will match with deposits to establish individual investment accounts. IDA funds can be used to start businesses, purchase cars or homes, pay college tuition, etc., but are not cash out accounts. The other two-thirds of the profits per year from the store will be shared equally among the worker-owners. The market was not open at the time of the site visit because of infrastructure and city permit delays, but it opened approximately 7 months after the visit.

The third supermarket program was the result of a community development corporation working with a chain supermarket to build a store on the site of an old automobile dealership. Developers had been interested in this location because of its position on a major city thoroughfare. In 1996, within a couple of years after planning started, the supermarket and other retail spaces in the plaza opened. The community development corporation was involved in the initial hiring of staff for the supermarket and offered a shuttle service for senior citizens and low-income residents. Currently, the store employs about 150 people, and about 80% of employees are neighborhood residents. The supermarket and other stores in the plaza have spurred other economic growth on property adjacent to or near to it. The market has been highly successful for the past 10 years, outperforming and exceeding expectations in terms of sales and customer satisfaction compared with other stores in the state and nearby areas. Though the primary focus of the initiative was economic revitalization of the neighborhood, one unintended consequence was increased access to a wider range of affordably priced food at a desirable market, in a neighborhood that had previously lacked any major grocery stores.

Another program visited had a different focus. A supermarket developed a navigation system that rated general foods, beverages, meats, poultry/seafood, dairy, nuts, baby foods, and fats and oils with zero, one star (good), two stars (better), or three stars (best). Stars appeared on unit price tags, scale labels, signs, and marketing materials. Items without stars did not meet the nutritional criteria for a star or have not been rated (bottled waters and other items with less than 5 calories per manufacturer's serving are not rated). The stars rating system is based on an evidence-based algorithm that was created by a nutrition science expert panel. The seven-member panel reviewed guidelines from DHHS, FDA, USDA, National Academies of Sciences, and the World Health Organization. The algorithm credit or debit points based the product's content on vitamins and minerals, dietary fiber, whole grains, trans fat, saturated fat, cholesterol, added sugar, and added sodium. The corporate officers and program staff at the supermarket recognize that the stars by themselves on item tags in the stores may not be effective, so they have integrated the use of dietitians, store tours, nutrition education classes, recipe rating, and consulting services. This raises awareness, educates, and encourages the use of rating system and healthier eating habits.

The neighborhood food watch aims to empower community members to improve the quality of foods sold in their neighborhood stores. Staff members describe the initiative as a social marketing campaign, as it is designed first to raise consumer awareness of what should be expected in terms of quality fresh produce and meats, and then to encourage consumers to advocate for their neighborhood stores to provide that level of quality. Residents are asked to complete a Store Quality Checklist each time they shop in a supermarket. Program staff also ask stores to agree to a list of standards of quality, which include: top-quality fresh fruit and vegetable selections; quality meat selections; fresh nonfat and low-fat dairy products; 100% whole grain breads and the like; limited products with saturated and trans fats; no perishable foods past their expired dates; fresh foods and demonstrating their use in nutritious recipes; placing healthier products in high-visibility locations; keeping the inside and outside of the store clean and safe and providing professional service; and ensuring competitive yet affordable pricing that was standardized among local stores of that chain.

The project team also conducted an EA of a program related to increasing access to healthier foods in the corner store setting by increasing the availability of items such as 1% milk and fruits and vegetables. The program goal was to establish corner stores as a venue for buying healthy foods. Corner stores—small retail shops, convenience stores, or bodegas that typically sell liquor and tobacco—were appropriate targets because of their prevalence and proximity in urban neighborhoods. They are often the only available food source for residents without access to a car.

In addition to working with store owners to stock healthier items, program staff members also conducted outreach and education in local schools, day care centers, and WIC centers to raise awareness about the availability of milk and produce at corner stores and to promote healthy eating. Program staff also worked to expand the program to other neighborhoods. During the pilot of the corner store program, store owners were required to offer a discount on 1% and skim milk as a promotion to attract consumers. As the program rolled out to more corner stores in the area, owners were not asked to discount their merchandise of healthier products because program staff did not want to place a financial burden on participants. According to program staff, it appeared that store owners were beginning to view healthy food and fresh produce as a new market opportunity, with a potential for profit. The small size of corner stores limited the range of products that the store could sell, and many stores did not have adequate space for fresh produce. Furthermore, owners of small stores had limited refrigerator space or understanding of how to store perishables. Program staff members worked to find creative solutions to these barriers. Several possible solutions were considered to attract funding to help upgrade the refrigeration systems of corner stores. Those solutions included the use of business improvement loans or grants through the city council, chamber of commerce, or local representatives and loans, grants, business advice, and technical assistance from private funders to existing stores.

Farmers Markets

The farmers market programs we examined were designed to increase the purchase of fresh fruits and vegetables among the low-income population by accepting electronic benefit transfer (EBT) and other food assistance benefits. The programs promoted the markets and advocated for supportive farmers market policies. One program connected farmers with schools, restaurants, hospitals, and retailers. Farmers market programs offered nutrition education such as cooking demonstrations and recipe distribution. One program we examined was a unique incentive program in which individuals were provided an additional \$2 to use after purchasing at least \$5 worth of produce with their EBT. Another program partnered with a produce distributor who sold produce at the wholesale price and delivered it directly to community-based organizations, which in turn offered the fresh produce for sale at various locations in the neighborhood.

From the EAs of five farmers markets, we learned that recipients of food assistance programs used the markets to purchase more fresh fruits and vegetables. Data from some of the programs indicate sizable EBT sales and redemption rates of vouchers at some farmers markets. For example, during 2007, EBT sales totaled more than $1,300 and WIC sales totaled nearly $3,000 at one farmers market. At one site, a growing customer base resulted in expansion from a farm stand managed by one person to a market with 10 farmer-vendors and approximately 750 customers per week. That farmers market program continually sought to add farmers markets in low-income neighborhoods. While it was plausible that the acceptance of EBT and WIC vouchers at farmers markets increased access to fresh fruits and vegetables, thereby increasing the purchase and consumption of healthier foods, one site visitor noted that it was less plausible that farmers markets alone decreased the prevalence of childhood obesity. It is unclear to what extent the purchase of fruits and vegetables translated to children eating healthier. Also, the role of farmers markets in preventing obesity appeared limited because they typically take place once a week; in many parts of the country they are only available from late spring through early fall. However, all site visitors agreed that the farmers markets provided fresh produce to communities that might otherwise not have had access to it, and this may have contributed to improving the eating habits of children and youths in low-income families.

Program staff reported that customers commonly expressed thoughts that "it's too hard," "too much trouble," or "too expensive" to shop for and prepare fresh food. Many of the ideas for encouraging the purchase of healthy foods in supermarkets and corner stores can also be implemented at farmers markets: food and cooking demonstrations; sample taste testings; and dissemination of information on how to select, store, and cook with healthy ingredients. Program staff also expressed that farmers markets have a reputation for being expensive, but many times there is little difference in the price of quality produce between farmers markets and other venues. Furthermore, in neighborhoods that do not have a full-service supermarket, farmers markets may be the only option for purchasing fresh fruits and vegetables. Activities to disseminate information about EBT and WIC or senior citizen voucher acceptance may encourage more customers to shop at farmers markets. To attract neighborhood residents who receive food assistance, some farmers markets used readily accessible, low-cost methods such as hanging banners and posters to advertise the acceptance of food assistance options. Program staff and market managers noted that they would like to increase this type of advertising. One program demonstrated that providing incentives—such as an additional $2 to use after purchasing at least $5 worth of produce—may be a worthwhile way to encourage more fruit and vegetable consumption by EBT recipients. Program staff cited a 40% redemption rate of its coupons.

Restaurants

Four of the five restaurant programs we examined had similar activities that focused on outreach to and recruitment of restaurants and the promotion of healthier menu options in local family owned restaurants (though in one program, chain restaurants such as McDonald's and Quizno's also participated). Restaurant program staff members were flexible in adapting the original project design to incorporate new ideas that were more appropriate for specific settings. For example, one restaurant program was adapted from its original setting in a suburban, middle-income population to an urban, low-income setting. Initially, program staff encouraged restaurant owners to add healthy items to their menus. Cooking classes were organized with a popular local chef to teach healthy cooking techniques (e.g., using spices and herbs instead of salt; grilling foods instead of frying; use of whole-wheat bread instead of white bread; and using low-fat milk instead of whole milk).

Three programs relied on comparative analysis of menu items to determine the healthier options. Only one program conducted nutritional analysis of menu items. To determine if the selected items met the eligibility criteria, the program required restaurant owners to submit their recipes for nutritional analysis (e.g., calories, total fat, cholesterol, sodium, protein, calcium, and iron). For most restaurants, the nutrition analysis of menu items is conducted at a discounted rate. However, depending upon how the restaurant was recruited into the program, the cost may be partially or fully subsidized. In most cases, only minor modifications to submitted recipes were needed to meet the program's eligibility criteria. Rarely was a new dish added to the menu in order to meet the nutritional requirements.

Similar in concept was the citywide calorie labeling policy requiring food service establishments (with 15 or more locations throughout the country to post calorie information prominently on menu boards and menus. Those establishments must post calorie information on all menu boards and menus where there is a price, food items displayed for sale with food item tags, any other list or pictorial display of a food item or items and price(s) posted, and menu boards or adjacent stanchions at or prior to the point of ordering for drive-through windows. Calorie information must be posted so that it clearly identifies the number of calories for each menu item; is clear and conspicuous, in close proximity to the relevant menu item; and is printed in a font and format that is at least as prominent as the name or price of the menu item. Food service establishments are expected to base the calorie content value on a verifiable analysis of the menu item, which may include laboratory testing, use of nutrient databases, or any other reliable method of analysis. Calorie counts are rounded off to the nearest 10 calories for counts above 50 and to the nearest 5 calories for counts at or below 50. The requirement is enforced by the city's department of health, who may issue citations for violations (fines between $200 to $2,000, with penalty amounts increasing for repeat inspections). Violations are also posted on the health department's restaurant inspection Web site, although they do not count toward the restaurant's inspection score. The local restaurant association has resisted this policy, and litigation has been one significant challenge to its implementation. The restaurant association filed a lawsuit in U.S. District Court claiming that the city's new ordinance was preempted by Federal law and, more broadly, that it violated the First Amendment. After several rounds of hearings and revisions to the calorie labeling proposal, the policy finally went into effect in April 2008.

Restaurant programs had varying degrees of fidelity among their participating sites; that is, sites did not all adhere to program design and were not uniform in their implementation of core components. For example, one restaurant program had 15 restaurants in the area that signed a commitment letter and agreed to highlight the healthier options on their menus. Several model restaurants did everything that was asked of them (display the program's decal on the door; display menu boards and posters highlighting the baked, steamed, and grilled items; and allow for data collection through observational counts). However, some restaurants were less dedicated to the program and did not display menu boards and posters and made little effort to provide or highlight healthier options for patrons. Interviews with restaurant owners revealed that the key reasons they continue with the program are because they receive free publicity—and increased patronage—and because participation does not require much effort on their part.

V. DISCUSSION

Plausibility

The food access programs we examined were based on the idea that efforts to increase access to affordable, nutritious food can have a positive outcome on health status.

For 12 of the 16 programs, site visitors reported that it was plausible that such interventions could have an impact on increasing access to healthier foods and thereby improving diet. In other words, the links between program components and expected outcomes are appropriate and plausible based on logic or available theory. As the availability of healthy foods increases, it likely plays an important role in determining a person's diet and risk of related chronic diseases. Changes in the environment, such as the opening of a supermarket or the availability of skim milk in restaurants, can improve dietary habits at the individual level and also at a population level. Increased access to healthy foods, combined with increased consumer awareness and nutrition education, will enable families to make healthier food choices. For the remaining three programs, site visitors specifically noted that they felt that the link between the intervention and prevention of childhood obesity was less plausible. The programs held promise as part of a larger, comprehensive, multipronged strategy to combat obesity, and it was not entirely plausible that the intervention alone will affect eating behaviors. Site visitors only mentioned the need for a more comprehensive approach for two programs, but we acknowledge that it is true for all programs. These programs would better impact health outcomes and contribute to preventing obesity as part of a larger, comprehensive effort than they would as stand-alone programs.

The theory that increasing access to healthier foods will impact obesity is plausible, though several site visitors noted that it is also important to increase consumer awareness of and consumer demand for healthier foods. Activities to increase access to healthy foods through these venues need to be carried out together with other activities, such as consumer education and health promotion. One of the most common challenges cited by programs was the need for more outreach to raise awareness about their efforts: teaching the community how to shop for and prepare healthy meals; promoting the acceptance of EBT, WIC, and senior vouchers at farmers markets; and highlighting the availability of healthier options at restaurants. Consumer demand is a key ingredient for all these programs, and extensive marketing is needed. As one program staff member noted, effective marketing can be done through radio commercials, flyers, and promotions at community events, senior centers, and schools. That strategy is applicable to all programs, regardless of venue.

Feasibility

All but one program were rated as feasible; that is, the interventions were likely to be implemented as designed. Program staff exhibited exemplary dedication, creativity, passion, and skills in carrying out program activities, demonstrating that it is feasible to implement such interventions in urban, low-income populations. Successful program implementation often required a site-level champion to resolve challenges and overcome barriers. A champion can be a creative market manager willing to design scrips/tokens for EBT redemption at a farmers market, a restaurant owner with diabetes who understands the importance of a healthy diet, or a local politician eager to revitalize his community with a full-service supermarket.

One supermarket program was not fully implemented during the time of the site visit. The scheduled store opening had changed several times, which clearly demonstrated that developing the market was a lengthy, challenging undertaking. However, site visitors noted several facilitators to its implementation, including community initiation and retained community involvement; strong, longterm partnerships with the local government, universities, and foundations; established infrastructure; and strong capacity of the umbrella organization.

Potential Impact

Nine of the 16 programs were reported to have a strong potential impact on the social and physical environment pertinent to healthy eating. By providing the opportunity to purchase healthier foods, those interventions have potential for impact on the social environment through community building, empowerment, partnerships, economic revitalization, and the physical environment. Two restaurant programs were reported to have some potential for impact on greater access to healthier food, contingent upon several conditions including program sustainability, compliance to program components from restaurants, and direct consumer marketing.

Three programs were reported to have limited potential impact because of lack of consumer demand for healthier options, limited capacity of small businesses, limited hours of operation, and limited reach to households in low-income areas. Although issues with feasibility of implementation needed to be resolved, site visitors acknowledged that the programs have potential for improving access to healthy food if the barriers to implementation could be overcome.

Evaluation Capacity of Programs

Program staff collected various types of data that can be used for process evaluation, to describe how the program was implemented, and to monitor program implementation. Those data sources will be useful for identifying changes to ensure that the program operates as planned according to the logic model and also for program improvement. Programs relied on surveys, observational data, sales transaction data, and anecdotes from customers and suppliers (farmers, restaurants) and distributors (market managers, restaurant staff). Current data collection efforts include customer surveys, farmer/owner/operator surveys, customer/item counts, EBT sales, supermarket sales, and redemption of coupons and vouchers.

Site visitors suggested data that were not collected but may be useful for further evaluation purposes: customer surveys of food selection, food preparation, and dollars spent on purchasing produce; attendance at nutrition education events at farmers markets; assessment of owners' and customers' knowledge and behavior; purchases of healthier items by location; and surveys or focus groups about attitudes toward healthy eating. Expert panel members noted that the presence of healthier foods in the home increases children's consumption of them, so data on purchasing patterns may be extrapolated to behavior.

Many of these programs were located in minority and immigrant communities. Another overall challenge with data collection was obtaining information from people who speak different languages (e.g., Spanish, Hmong, Russian). Programs attempted to minimize the challenges by hiring staff who reflected the community.

The implementation of environmental interventions to increase access to healthier foods is pioneering because no model or blueprint is available to guide the way. The work presents many new questions and activities, and it brings together individuals from different sectors. Evaluation of the long-term effects—the purchase and consumption of healthier foods, improved nutrition, and improved health outcomes—is complex and requires resources, including staff with evaluation capacity, time, and money for longitudinal data collection. However, as the project team has seen, it is possible to build the foundation needed to make such evaluation possible through a common understanding of program goals and continued data collection.

Many sites expressed interest in learning more about other programs in the field. Knowledge sharing among organizations and groups seeking to increase access to healthy foods would be a helpful step to building empirical evidence.

Also, a research network devoted to food access would provide researchers an opportunity to share findings and discuss issues, options, and results.

Potential evaluation questions for each type of program, as identified by site visitors and the expert panel, are discussed in the following section.

Potential Evaluation Designs

Supermarkets and Corner Stores

The current data sources for the supermarket/corner store programs we visited included:

- Inventory of store merchandise
- Supermarket sales data

One possible evaluation design offered by the expert panel was to compare supermarket interventions to those of farmers markets in a cluster analysis and observe what differences the product selection, location, and seasonality have on customers. Another possible evaluation is a prestudy/poststudy examining food outlets in the area where a new supermarket is proposed. Possible measures would include transit time, food purchases, and cost (using receipts). It may also be helpful to study the economic impact of placing a new supermarket in an area where one does not exist. Related studies may explore the consequences of new supermarket placement for local small businesses.

Potential evaluation questions for supermarket and corner store programs include:

- What is the impact of the presence of a full-service supermarket on residents' diets?
- What are customers purchasing at supermarkets?
- At corner stores, are customers purchasing healthier options, such as 1% milk and fresh produce?
- How are foods being prepared after purchase?
- What is the economic impact of a new supermarket in the area?

Farmers Markets

The current data sources for the farmers market programs we visited included:

- Surveys with customers
- Surveys with farmers
- Surveys with market managers
- Ad hoc customer counts (hourly or daily)
- Farmer sales
- EBT sales
- Voucher sales
- Coupon redemption
- Anecdotes from customers and farmers
- Distribution of nutrition and health promotion materials
- Focus group and exit interviews with consumers

One farmers market incentive program had an innovative method to track the origin of coupon distribution. A code linked the coupon to where it was distributed (at a community-based organization or a particular farmers market). The program also collected information on any additional dollar amounts spent in conjunction with the incentive coupon—whether there were additional cash purchases, EBT purchases, or credit card purchases.

Members of the expert panel felt that evaluation designs best suited to answer the sentinel questions for farmers markets include a cluster design with a series of case studies or a multisite, multilevel comparison. They offered the following questions for evaluation of farmers market programs:

- What is the role of farmers markets in overall food shopping?
- What is the impact of the presence of farmers markets on residents' diets? Do farmers markets change food preferences or eating behaviors?
- Who is shopping at farmers markets (demographics, socioeconomic status)? What percentage of customers at markets are low income?
- How many people are using EBT/WIC/senior citizen vouchers at farmers markets?
- Where is the best venue for distributing incentives or vouchers for farmers markets? How should they be distributed to ensure redemption?
- How do farmers markets interact with social determinants of health?

- Do farmers markets create economic opportunities for the community? What is the business case to be made? How will supermarkets and other grocery stores respond to farmers markets in the long term?
- A major contextual factor for farmers markets is seasonality. How much time must a market be open in order to truly increase access to and purchase of healthier foods?
- What is the best way to influence the price of products at farmers markets?

Restaurants

The current data sources for the restaurant programs we visited included:

- Observational counts of total sales
- Observational counts of healthier items ordered
- Anecdotes from customers and restaurant staff
- Copies of menus and ingredient lists, where available
- Focus groups and interviews with restaurant owners

For the calorie labeling initiative specifically, expert panel members suggested that it be evaluated in a cluster design during implementation in several cities. The panelists explained that it would be particularly valuable to study the initiative as it was adopted in other locations. The panel expressed enthusiasm for the idea of doing a cluster evaluation, which would allow for comparative multiple baseline measures. The panel noted their hope that any lessons learned from local evaluations of calorie labeling initiatives would inform national policy.

Case studies would be helpful for addressing restaurant programs because of the limited information in this area. Case studies could be useful in addressing such questions as how the program got started, and what it takes to sustain it. The expert panel posited other evaluation questions.

- What is the effect of offering healthier menu options on customer purchases?
- What is the financial impact of changes on small, family-owned restaurants (limiting free refills on sodas and sugar-sweetened beverages; changes in cooking practices; limiting portion sizes; cost of healthier items; storage of fresh fruits and vegetables)?

- Are customers substituting items with healthier alternatives when given a choice (e.g., whole- wheat bread over white bread, water over soda, fruit over cake)?

VI. Recommendations and Lessons Learned

We acknowledge the strengths of the programs and provide recommendations and lessons learned to inform future activities. While recommendations and lessons learned are categorized according to the type of program or policy (supermarkets and corner stores, farmers markets, and restaurants), there are communalities that can be generalized for all programs.

Supermarkets and Corner Stores

Leverage Available Resources

Renovating, developing, or attracting supermarkets and grocery stores to urban areas required tremendous financial resources and community commitment. These initiatives were often coordinated by local nonprofit organizations in partnership with community investment groups, community development corporations, and local leadership (e.g., mayor, city council member, State assembly person, county department of health). Because financing and capital gaps were often barriers to supermarket development, the program staff worked to meet the financing needs of store owners who planned to operate in underserved communities where infrastructure costs and credit needs could not be filled solely by conventional financial institutions. This initiative was supported by strong partnerships with a community development bank, an active community-based organization, State legislators, and funding leveraged from tax credits for economic development. The building of supermarkets in low-income areas was feasible because community members and staff built a strong case for it, with evidence presented about an important public health and economic need to partners, funders, and the community. By incorporating an economic stimulus package into a public health intervention, this supermarket initiative was able to bring in legislators and public policymakers, resulting in the securing of millions of dollars in funding. Program staff members demonstrated to politicians and communities the benefits of the proposed initiative. Those interested in replicating the effort will need to develop strong partnerships, secure financial resources, and broaden the vision to attract nontraditional public health partners. As these programs have demonstrated, it can be done. Tapping new sources for capital costs will be vital to ensuring success; some possible avenues include community reinvestment funds, tax breaks, State grants, interest-free loans, and private investments. While the staff of the food cooperative initiative encountered long delays with the actual buildout and completion of the market (because of issues with the general contractor, rules for securing permits, and problems with space configuration), they eventually opened the market. The initiative staff plan to document the experience with developing the market and discuss their resolutions. Their in-depth report could be a useful way to inform the project as well as other underserved urban communities interested in developing and operating a locally owned supermarket.

Increase Marketing Efforts of Healthy Foods

Site visitors noted that although the supermarkets and corner stores had increased access to greater food diversity (through lowered food prices and reduced transportation costs), shoppers did not necessarily buy healthy items. The stores tried to address that disparity through citywide campaigns and marketing activities. At one site, a citywide campaign encouraged consumers to purchase skim milk and fruits and vegetables. Stores were also asked to display educational posters about healthy eating. Because taste is one of the most important factors in determining purchase, one strategy to help people choose healthy food was to offer free samples at the point of sale. Other ideas to encourage consumers to buy healthier foods included prominent shelf space and display of healthy items in stores and nutrition education classes to provide shopping and menu planning guidance. Displaying information about the food pyramid, label reading, choosing and storing produce, and seasonal guides to fruits and vegetables may also help to encourage the purchase of healthier foods. Such activities can help to create positive attitudes toward healthy eating.

Use the Nutrition Environment Measures Survey in Stores

Program staff of the supermarket and corner store programs may consider using the Nutrition Environment Measures Survey in Stores (NEMS-S) tool, a tested and validated instrument to systematically review markets (Glanz et al. 2007). The tool can be found online at http://www.sph.emory.edu/NEMS/NEMS_S_Detailed.pdf. However, the use of NEMS-S may require a level of expertise and resources beyond the reach of some program staff. Other user-friendly tools for assessing the consumer food environment include the Baltimore Health Eating Zones Food Source Checklist, which assesses store characteristics and availability of key healthy foods, and the Food Stores Survey, which assesses the availability of a few selected healthy foods in convenience stores and grocery stores in low-income neighborhoods (Ohri-Vachaspati & Leviton, in press).

Partner with Others

The corner store approach is promising because it brings healthy food into existing stores, avoiding the challenges of adding full-service supermarkets in neighborhoods where space is limited and major funding needs to be secured. To decrease the costs of buying produce from distributors, corners markets could collaborate with local farmers markets and working directly with growers to acquire fresh and locally grown produce. Some major chain supermarkets are experimenting with opening corner stores, therefore it may be an opportunity for existing corner stores to consider initiating partnerships with major chain supermarkets. The supermarket could buy produce and other goods and store, deliver, and provide the products to the corner stores. With this arrangement, corner stores could benefit from the buying power of the larger market.

It is important to view grocery stores and supermarkets as important contributors to neighborhood quality of life through improved food access and, by extension, potentially improved nutrition. Strong community partnerships can help stores to promote confidence among residents, and active involvement from the mayor, city planning commission, and economic development agencies can aid in developing the supermarket.

Farmers Markets

Synergize Efforts

One site visitor noted that the farmers market program she visited had several important strengths, including size, longevity, stability, growth, efficient use of constrained resources, and local and State policy support. The program was also situated within a mature, strong parent organization that has programmatic and evaluation resources. The availability of resources and ability to coordinate with programs to reduce the burdens of obesity produces synergy and ensures that activities are planned for a common goal. Those involved in the farmers markets programs and activities know the community, are respected, and have been successful in getting the community's buy-in.

Improve Social Health

In addition to improving physical health, farmers markets may also be a way to improve social health. Staff at three of the farmers market programs stated that they would also like the markets to be a destination—a safe, pleasant space where senior citizens, children, and families can interact with their neighbors. This perspective is important because it broadens the traditional scope and function of farmers markets. It is important to realize that these markets can provide a social opportunity, especially for low-income individuals with limited mobility.

Be Patient

Most farmers markets have limited funding. Some receive small grants from the city, school district, or other local organizations, and many rely on the farmer stall fees (which are usually minimal). Often, initiating a market requires market operators or managers to supply the upfront costs of promotion, licensing and insurance, equipment and supplies, and equipment storage. Farmers markets are financial endeavors that require time to grow and succeed; and it may not be reasonable to expect an immediate return on investment. One farmers market manager reported that it took 7 years for her market to simply break even. Startup costs and expenses for maintaining a business— particularly one in a low-income neighborhood—may be more than many small businesses can handle.

Use Local Volunteers

To mitigate the challenge of limited funds and therefore limited staffing, one farmers market used service learners (college students enrolled in a community service class) to volunteer and assist with the duties of running the market. Program staff may consider developing ways to sustain active relationships with neighborhood associations and other community groups. Program staff can recruit neighborhood leaders to manage or conduct nutrition education at the farmers market, train volunteers to perform some tasks, and work with neighborhood associations and supporters to develop and conduct enhanced outreach for the farmers markets. Such approaches would further enhance neighborhood cohesion.

Implementing EBT Acceptance Is Not Difficult

Interviewees noted the value of a committed site-level champion—usually the market manager— who completes the paperwork and tasks needed to initiate the acceptance of EBT. While these tasks are not difficult, they may take time, which has deterred many operators from accepting EBT. Site visitors from one program provided some common challenges to initiating the acceptance of EBT at farmers markets.

- Creation of a scrip. Outdoor food markets and produce stands do not usually have the electricity and telephone lines needed for all eligible food vendors to deal with EBTs. Therefore, many markets allow all eligible food vendors to sell eligible food products to EBT cardholders by setting up a central point of sale (POS) device to sell market scrips (wooden tokens representing a certain monetary value) to customers, who can then use them to shop in the market. EBT cards are debited at the central terminal, where customers receive the scrips to do their shopping among the various market vendors. The vendors are later reimbursed by the market management for the number of scrips they have collected. The system requires the market management to become authorized to accept EBT food benefits and to organize and promote the use of EBT cards at the market. The scrips typically are marked with the market's logo and a denomination.
- Application for an EBT permit. A farmers market interested in accepting EBT needs to designate an individual (e.g., market manager, board chair) to submit an application to USDA Food and Nutrition Services for a permit. USDA approves the application and forwards it to the State Department of Social Services (DSS) Electronic Benefits Transfer Unit. The department reviews the scrip package and arranges for telephone training. USDA approval takes 20 to 45 days, and the State DSS EBT approval can take up to 2 months. If approved, the State DSS office provides phone support to ensure that the market is capable and comfortable accepting EBT.
- Setting up a central POS. If a market does not have the electricity and telephone connections needed for individual vendors to deal with EBTs, they may set up a central POS device to sell market scrips to customers. The market manager, or a reliable delegate, must be present throughout the market's period of operation to facilitate this exchange with all customers.

As those farmers market programs have demonstrated, it is possible to implement and adopt EBT acceptance. The first step is to garner the market manager's buy-in about the benefits of accepting EBT cards and the positive impact of providing healthy produce to the community.

Restaurants

Attract More Participating Restaurants

Additional marketing efforts may encourage current owners to sustain participation and attract new restaurant owners. It may be helpful if program staff use their success stories to let other restaurant owners know about the benefits of the program. For example, if a restaurant owner agrees to be a program champion, flyers with his or her picture and words of endorsement that also speak to the economic benefits of participation could be created and given to other restaurants as part of the recruitment effort. The program could also be advertised and recruit owners by placing ads in local community newspapers.

Align Health Goals With Business Goals

Staff members learned that it took more time than they originally thought to work with restaurants and negotiate a set of changes to their menus and restaurant environments. In addition, working with for-profit businesses was a new experience for many program staff members. While a priority of businesses may be to increase profits, it is possible to align health goals with business goals. Restaurant programs found that forming partnerships with businesses, financing organizations, and media outlets can be beneficial because they provide funding sources, communication avenues, and skill sets from different sectors. For many family-owned small restaurants, it is difficult to compete against fast-food chains in the area. Programs should consider using the rich resources available in their communities (e.g., local chamber of commerce, community health centers, advocacy organizations, local radio stations, schools, and, where relevant, CDC Prevention Research Centers) to promote the businesses or assist with program development. Program staff and site visitors noted that the proprietors of family-owned businesses, many of them restaurant owners, were not trained on how to successfully run a business, especially one with such low profit margins. Providing such information to owners in a user-friendly format could reap several benefits: it could function as an incentive for owner participation, especially if it were free or low cost and not time consuming; and it could increase the likelihood that a restaurant would stay in business (and stay in the program) while contributing to the economic development of the neighborhood. It may be possible for program staff to work with some of their community partners or other local community economic development agencies to provide information to restaurant owners via referrals, trainings, or other forms of technical assistance.

Brand and Market the Program

The four restaurant programs have branded their campaign, creating a logo and window decals to show which restaurants offer healthier options. In addition, program staff created table tents and menu boards to feature healthier menu items identified by criteria established with a registered dietitian. Because branding is a key component of any consumer product, incorporating key social marketing principles into the program may help to strengthen those restaurant program components. The National Cancer Institute's Making Health Communication Programs Work (commonly referred to as the Pink Book), one of the leading texts in health communication, is based on a social marketing framework. (The online version of this publication is available at http://www.cancer Tools of Change is another excellent online source for information on community-based social marketing (http://www.toolsofchange.com/English/ firstsplit.asp). In marketing and describing the program, staff should also consider how the concept of healthier is framed. Emphasis on healthfulness may only appeal to a small population; instead, promoting great taste, quality, and convenience may be more appealing to the general population.

Understand the Community

The staff at restaurant programs also noted the importance of understanding one's own community in order to determine the appropriate intervention or strategy. The staff of one program acknowledged that it needed to hire Spanish-speaking staff to recruit restaurants in a predominantly Latino community. Because of her cultural background, this staff member was able to relate and communicate with the restaurant owners and managers, thereby gaining their trust and buy-in.

Be Flexible

Many of the small, family-owned businesses in the low-income neighborhood operated with very low profit margins and had limited capacity for refrigeration and storage; consequently, the owners were wary of offering items such as fresh fruits or vegetables if they could not be sold quickly. To address these concerns, program staff shifted their focus from adding healthy options to the menu to highlighting items already on the menu that could be considered healthier options. This new approach made it easier for restaurants to participate in the program because they were not required to change the way they did business. The programs are replicable, but they may need to be tailored to appeal to a specific community or target audience. One size does not fit all, especially for family-owned restaurants, and program staff members implemented creative solutions for individual restaurants to address their challenges.

Educate Consumers

Restaurant programs may consider devoting resources (time and staff) to activities aimed at educating residents about what healthy options are available, as well as the importance and benefits of choosing such options when shopping and dining out. Without this type of education, it may be difficult for the program to achieve both its long-term goals and expected outcomes. Site visitors noted that without sufficient consumer demand, it may also be difficult for the programs to grow to the scale that is needed to bring about the desired changes. Similar to the supermarkets, corner stores, and farmers markets, restaurants can use taste testing, food coupons, and other direct marketing efforts to increase the program's visibility. More of these activities will continue to help raise awareness and build support among community members. For the calorie-labeling initiative, several interviewees noted that they would like to put more efforts on advertising to increase the public's understanding of the calorie numbers posted and that the total number of calories the average person needs in a day is only 2,000. Greater awareness is an important aspect of ensuring that people will improve their overall diet.

VII. Limitations of Methods

We have attempted to synthesize what we have learned about food access programs based on site visitors' reports from the EAs. The methodology has several limitations. First, given our bird's-eye view of these programs, our findings may not apply to every program, although we acknowledge that the ones we examined supported health promotion and obesity prevention. Second, because programs differed in venue, scope, and level of implementation, aggregate themes did not tell the whole story. In addition, we examined three very different types of food access programs. Whenever appropriate, we provided separate findings for supermarkets/corner stores, farmers markets, and restaurants. Third, the small sample size made generalizations inappropriate. However, we gained a feel for the important issues in food access programs, which we attempted to convey. Fourth, the data we used to compile this synthesis primarily came from site visitors' reports. While site visitors were provided a template for reporting, the amount of information and type of information in the reports varied, making comparisons across all the programs difficult. Site visitors were asked to provide additional or clarifying information in the reports when possible; differences may be due to the unavailability or lack of data from some programs.

VIII. Conclusion

The project team learned from the EA site visits that local governments, nonprofit organizations, community groups, and businesses were working to increase the availability of healthier foods, particularly in low-income and underserved neighborhoods. Such efforts encouraged the purchase of fruits and vegetables at farmers markets and expanded healthier food options at local grocery stores, supermarkets, and restaurants. The large number of nominations received and the high level of interest in participating in this EA process were evidence that many promising community-level interventions were being implemented. Staff, partners, and site visitors perceived these programs as exciting endeavors that had the potential to help prevent childhood obesity.

Appendix A. Description of Selection Criteria

Description of Selection Criteria

Potential Impact. The intervention appears to have potential for impact on the social or physical environment pertinent to healthy eating and active living—and ultimately on the target individual behaviors. Potential impact is assessed based on the intervention's conceptual logic and other pertinent characteristics, such as intensity and duration. Estimate of impact is based on "face value," program documents, and brief expert input from funding organization staff and contractors, and other experts who know the intervention but are independent from it.

Innovativeness. Intervention is new or different or a significant variation on an existing promising intervention. Emphasis on innovativeness may be mitigated if the intervention represents a type or category of intervention that is prevalent in the field and/or of particular interest to Robert Wood Johnson Foundation and collaborating organizations.

Reach to Target Population. The likelihood or actual evidence that the intervention will achieve participation (and even retention and completion) by the target population (i.e., approximately what percentage of the target population is likely to or actually does participate in or is "reached" in some other way by the intervention).

Acceptability to Stakeholders. The potential or actual evidence that the intervention is acceptable and even attractive to pertinent collaborators, gatekeepers, and other necessary groups, such as schools, businesses, government agencies, grassroots groups, and so forth.

Feasibility of Implementation. The likelihood that the intervention as designed can be fully implemented given the clarity of its goals, objectives, and strategies; complexity and leadership requirements; financial and other costs; and training and supervision requirements. If evidence exists regarding program implementation, then the extent to which the intervention "on paper" has been fully and faithfully implemented and the degree of difficulty in achieving implementation.

Feasibility of Adoption. The potential for similar sites/entities to adopt the intervention.

Intervention Sustainability. The likelihood that the intervention can continue over time without special resources or extraordinary leadership.

Generalizability. The degree to which the intervention demonstrates or has potential to be adapted for other populations and settings.

Staff/Organizational Capacity. Sponsoring organization and staff have the capacity to participate fully in a brief assessment, learn from it, and further develop the intervention.

Appendix B. Logic Model

Problem Statement

A healthy diet contributes to obesity prevention. A common barrier to maintaining a healthy diet among children in families with low incomes is limited access to healthy food choices in terms of availability, affordability, and quality.

INPUTS	ACTIVITIES	OUTPUTS	SHORT-TERM OUTCOMES (~ 1 to 3 years)	INTERMEDIATE OUTCOMES (~ 3 to 5 years)	LONG-TERM OUTCOMES (~ 4 to 6 years)	GOAL
• Fresh produce and/or other healthy food options • Partners (community, private, government) • Financing • Personnel, including staff and volunteers • Materials and equipment (e.g., promotional flyers, cash registers, EBT machines)	• Promotion and marketing of farmers' market, supermarket, or restaurant • Make fresh produce and/or other healthier food options available • Raise consumer awareness about healthier food options • Nutrition education/ cooking demonstrations • Accept food assistance such as EBT, WIC, Senior Coupons (for farmers' markets and supermarkets only)	• Number or proportion of produce/healthier food options • Number of nutrition education sessions • Number of promotional events or materials displayed • Number of EBT machines available (for farmers' market and supermarkets only)	• Availability of quality and affordable healthier options in the community • Increased access to affordable fresh produce and/or other healthy food options for low-income families with children	• Increased awareness of healthier food options in the community • Increased purchases of fresh produce and/or other healthy food options among low-income families with children • Improved, positive attitudes toward healthy eating	• Increased consumption of healthy food options among individuals in low-income families with children • Increased sales for supermarkets and corner stores, farmers' markets, restaurants	• Contribute to improving the access to and availability of healthier foods in low-income communities • Improved health outcomes due to reduction in diet-related diseases
Data source to document accomplishment	Attendance records at activities, documentation of protocol, nutrition education materials	Attendance records at activities	Inventory records at restaurants and markets; observational counts of customers	Customer purchase data over a period of time, inventory records, sales data, customer surveys	Customer purchase data over a period of time; consumer surveys; consumer interviews	

Appendix C. Descriptions of Food Access Programs that Participated in an Evaluability Assessment

Program	Target Audience	Main Program Components	Expected Outcomes Supermarkets/Corner	Goals of Program Stores	Plausibility	Feasibility	Potential Impact
Supermarket Initiative Number 1	Low-income communities	• Advocate at State and local levels for funding to build or renovate new supermarkets • Outreach to promote program to communities and store operators • Obtain community buy-in and establish task force • Create financing or distribution mechanism to help establish or assist supermarkets in underserved areas	• Increase in number of supermarkets opening and operating in underserved areas • Increase in purchase and consumption of fresh produce and/or other healthier food options • Supermarkets meeting needs of consumers and meeting profitability objectives • Increased development of other small enterprises in the area	• Contribute to improving the access to fresh foods • Improve health outcomes by reducing diet-related disease, increasing social capital, and improving well-being • Economic development	Plausible	Feasible, though it may require strong program staff and resources	Strong potential impact on physical and economic environment of underserved areas by providing access to supermarkets and creating job opportunities

Supermarket Initiative Number 2	Low-income families, especially those with children	• Obtain financing for supermarket • Secure physical space • Hire and train worker- owners Develop and offer a cooperative economic investment program for area residents • Implement nutrition education activities in the market	• Increased access to a variety of affordable, fresh produce and other healthy foods • Increased employment and job skills for area residents • Increased purchases and consumption of healthier food	• Launch and operate a large, locally owned cooperative supermarket with a nutrition education center • Increased economic development of the neighborhood	Plausible	Feasible, though market has experienced various delaysnin opening and operation	Strong potential impact
Supermarket Initiative Number 3	Low-income neighborhood with a historically high unemployment rate Considered the most distressed area of the city	• Obtain financing for building and maintaining supermarket • Hire and train neighborhood staff • Marketing and development of the supermarket	• Increased access to food • Increased purchasing of healthier food in the neighborhood • Increased pride in the community • Increased property value • Increased employment opportunities	• Improve the social and economic well- being of the neighborhood • Maintain an inviting, well-managed, affordable, accessible option for purchasing food	Plausible	Feasible; store has been in existence for more than a decade	Strong potential impact, though the focus has not traditionally been on childhood obesity

Appendix C (Continued).

Program	Target Audience	Main Program Components	Expected Outcomes Supermarkets/Corner	Goals of Program Stores	Plausibility	Feasibility	Potential Impact
Supermarket Navigation Rating System	All potential consumers of the chain supermarket and its affiliates Other supermarkets interested in using the system in their stores	• Create algorithm and maintain database of rated items • Display product scores • Build awareness of program through health fairs, community events, and partnerships with doctors' offices, schools, and health department • Market the rating system to consumers and also to other supermarkets	• Increase consumers' purchases of nutritious items • Loyal customers continue and/or increase purchases of highly rated items as part of a nutritious diet • Adoption of the rating system by other supermarkets • Increased number of products reformulated by manufacturers to be more nutritious	• Establish the item-rating system as the premier nutritional navigation system • Improve the nutrition of consumers • Improve the health and wellness of communities	Plausible	Feasible	Strong potential impact, especially if this system becomes available in stores nationwide manufacturers reformulate their products to be more nutritious
Supermarket Neighborhood Watch Program	Low-income communities Children and youth in low-income African American families	• Discuss with neighborhood stores the Standards of Quality • Raise community expectations for	• Increased community members' expectations for healthy, quality foods Participating stores offer increased	• Improve access to and availability of healthier foods among residents in the area	Plausible; however, the link between the program and prevention of	Feasible, though having stores sign the Standards of Quality Agreement	Potential impact on increased community expectations and relationship-building with local retailers

		healthful foods and quality food retail environment	selection of fresh produce, top- grade meats, low-fat dairy, unexpired items, and whole grains at affordable and standardized prices • Increased consumption of healthier food options		childhood obesity is less direct and it is not certain that stores will signify-cantly improve the quality of their offeri-ngs to the degree that it will impact residents' health	may be less feasible; there is resistance from food retailers about the legal impacts of a binding agreement	
Corner Store Initiative	Low-income families	• Deliver 1% milk toolkits and provide education to bodegas • Negotiate with milk distributors to provide discounts on 1% milk to bodega owners • Distribute promotional materials to WIC, day care, and health centers	• Increased number of bodegas stocking 1% milk • Community members understand the importance of switching from whole milk to 1% milk • Increased sales of 1% milk	• Increase access to food for the community • Decrease the incidence of obesity and diet-related diseases, including diabetes and heart disease	Less plausible	Feasible, though it requires strong community partnerships	Strong potential impact on physical and social environment, through partnerships and community building

Appendix C (Continued).

Program	Target Audience	Main Program Components	Expected Outcomes Supermarkets/Corner	Goals of Program Stores	Plausibility	Feasibility	Potential Impact
Farmers Market Number 1	• Low-income residents in the city and its neighboring areas • Senior citizens	• Recruit and retain farmers • Promote markets • Provide nutrition education • Make EBT machines available to farmers and retailers • Advocate for supportive farmers market policies	• Increased availability of fresh produce for neighborhood householdsIncreased knowledge among consumers about preparation of fresh produce • Increased purchase and consumption of fresh fruits and vegetables • Sustainability of farmers markets	• Contribute to increased habitual consumption of fresh fruit and vegetables • Improve health by preventing obesity and diabetes	Less plausible	Feasible	Limited potential impact, due to seasonality of market and limited reach to low-income households
Farmers Market Number 2	• Low-income residents in the community • African American; Latino, Hmong, and Russian immigrants	• Provide culturally appropriate and locally grown produce at farmers markets • Promote farmers markets • Provide customer education, such as cooking demonstrations and nutrition classes	• Increased purchase and consumption of fresh fruits and vegetables • Increased consumption of healthier food options • Increased number of growers participating in farmers markets • Improved cooking and dietary habits • Increased community cohesion	• Contribute to improving the eating habits of low-income families	Plausible	Feasible	Strong potential impact on physical environment by providing access to fruits and vegetables for low-income families

		Make EBT, WIC, and senior vouchers acceptable at farmers markets					
Farmers Market Number 3	• Low-income residents • Hispanics • Other stakeholder audiences and community leaders, the media, economic advisers and decision makers, and health-professionals	• Provide nutrition education to patrons with FSNE eligibles • Collaborate with farmers market associations, agricultural organizations, and land use and hunger advocates • Research benefits, barriers, and best practices of farmers markets • Create a marketing campaign for farmers and residents • C onnect farmers with schools, restaurants, hospitals, and retailers	• Increased availability of fresh produce in the community • Increased purchase options for those with food assistance (EBT, WIC, and senior vouchers) • Increased consumption of fresh produce among residents in the community • Increased positive attitudes regarding healthy eating in the community • Commitment to accept EBT, WIC, and senior vouchers in farmers markets	• Reduce obesity, especially among children • Increase access to affordable, nutritious foods	Plausible	Feasible	Strong potential impact on physical environment by providing access to fruits and vegetables for low-income families

Appendix C (Continued).

Program	Target Audience	Main Program Components	Expected Outcomes Supermarkets/Corner	Goals of Program Stores	Plausibility	Feasibility	Potential Impact
		• Research benefits and how to overcome barriers of accepting food stamps and EBT cards					
Farmers Market Incentive Program	• Mothers from the WIC program • Low-income families	• Incentive program in which farmers markets provide an additional $2 to individuals who use $5 in food stamp (EBT) purchases • Promote the acceptance of EBT and Health Bucks by farmers markets • Promote the use of Health Bucks in low- income areas through community-based organizations,	• Increased awareness of the incentive program among residents • Increased redemption coupons • Increased purchase and consumption of fresh fruits and vegetables • Markets become community meeting places, strengthening community identity	• Expand access to healthy foods • Contribute to improving the eating habits of children and youth in low-income families	Plausible	Feasible	Potential impact on individual behavior and purchase patterns

		health promotion agencies, and faith-based organizations • Provide consumer education					
Produce Distribution Program	Low-income communities with high rates of childhood obesity Minor-ity populations	• Partner with a produce distributor who will sell produce at whole-sale prices and deliver directly to community-based organizations • Discount fresh produce market is held at community-based organization or Minority Health Promotion Centers	• Increased access to high-quality, affordable, and ethnically appropriate produce across the community • Increased purchase and consumption of fruits and vegetables • Increased knowledge, skills, and awareness regarding healthy eating behaviors	• Make access to fresh fruits and vegetables more convenient and affordable • Provide high-quality and ethnically appealing fruits and vegetables	Plausible	Feasible	Strong potential impact on physical environ-ment by chang-ing the food dis-tribution system

Appendix C (Continued).

Program	Target Audience	Main Program Components	Expected Outcomes Supermarkets/Corner	Goals of Program Stores	Plausibility	Feasibility	Potential Impact
Restaurant Program Number 1	Residents in the city, particularly African American and low-income residents	• Outreach to and recruitment of restaurants • Develop criteria for participation (nutrition-al and pricing criteria) • Provide technical assistance/work with restaurants to change menu in order to meet nutritional and pricing criteria • Develop program brand and promotional materials (logo, program designscheme, table tents, menu stickers, window decals, and brochures) • Display program logo in participating restaurants	• Increased patronage at restaurants participating in the program • Increased number of accessible restaurants in the program • Increased awareness among residents and interest in the program • Restaurant environment changes (e.g., changes in menu) • Increase the number of people going to a restaurant in the program • Increased number of people choosing healthier menu items at participating restaurants	• Create a healthier food environment in the city with the aim of reducing rates of cardiovascular disease	Plausible	Feasible; program has been adapted from its original model to be implem-ented in an urban, low-income setting	Limited potential impact due to lack of consumer demand

Restaurant Program Number 2	• Owners of family-owned restaurants • Residents in the area (primarily low- income African American and Hispanic)	• Outreach to and recruitment of restaurants • Promote and highlight healthier food options currently offered in local family-owned restaurants (e.g., steamed vegetables, baked chicken/fish, grilled meats, salads, 1% milk) • Develop and display promotional materials (window decal of program logo, menu boards, table tents, brochures) in restaurants	• Increased awareness of healthier food options at participating restaurants among area residents • Increased consumption of healthier food options among customers of participating restaurants • Improved positive attitudes regarding healthy eating in the community • Increased publicity and new catering opportunities for Restaurants • Sustained commitment to provide healthier food options among restaurant owners • Increased sales and profits	• Increase the availability and consumption of healthier options in local restaurants • Reduce the risks of developing heart disease and obesity-related morbidity	Plausible	Feasible; scope of program is manageable	Potential impact on physical envi-ronment by providing health-ier options in restaurants

Appendix C (Continued).

Program	Target Audience	Main Program Components	Expected Outcomes Supermarkets/Corner	Goals of Program Stores	Plausibility	Feasibility	Potential Impact
		• Conduct publicity events (taste testing, food festival, radio and local news promotion) to promote neighborhood restaurants					
Restaurant Program Number 3	• Restaurants, including chain fast-food establishments • Consumers and patrons of restaurants	• Recruit restaurants • Conduct menu analysis of items to feature as healthier options • Conduct in-store promotion of healthier options • Participate in public relations events (conferences, presentation)	• Increased awareness of healthier options at participating restaurants • Increased purchase of healthier options in restaurants • Increased consumption of fruits, vegetables, beans, and whole grains outside of the home	• Increase the number of healthy restaurant environments • Increase consumer demand for healthier options • Increase healthy eating • Reduce obesity and associated chronic diseases	Plausible	May be feasible, though program currently lacks staff time and resources	Limited potential impact currently; however, program may have impact if more staff time and resources are devoted to program implementation, evaluation, and direct consumer marketing

Restaurant Program Number 4	• Restaurant owners • Consumers and patrons of estaurants	• Recruit restaurants to participate • Assist restaurant to highlight healthier choices on menus, including menu analysis	• Increase awareness of healthier menu items in restaurants • Increase awareness of substitute, healthier ingredients and portion options in restaurants	• Improved nutritional/ dietary practices among families in the county	Plausible	Feasible	Some potential impact in improving food access for the community if program can be sustained and restaurant
		• Promote restaurants via the Internet, print, TV, radio media outlets, promotional activities	• Increase requests for substitutions • Increase patronage of restaurants and CS that provide healthier choices	• Contribution to decrease number of overweight children and rates of childhood obesity among families in the county			Compliance can be increased
Calorie Labeling Imitative	• Owners of restaurants with more than 15 locations nationwide • Residents in the area	• Citywide regulation requiring food service establishments to post the calorie content of menu items	• Consumers are more aware of calorie content • Restaurants change their offerings to make them healthier • National-level action requiring calorie labeling in chain restaurants across the country	Contribute to improving the food environment so that it is easier for customers to make healthier/lower calorie food and beverage choices	Plausible	Feasible	Strong potential impact on the environment relevant to healthy eating; requirement appears to en-courage restau-rants to make changes to their menu offerings to provide healthier options to consumers

References

Beaulac, J., Kristjansson, E. & Cummins, S. (2009). A systematic review of food deserts, 1966-2007. *Prevention of Chronic Disease*, *6(3)*, Retrieved August 5, 2009, from http://www.cdc.gov/pcd/issues 63.htm.

Block, J., Scribner, R. & DeSalvo, K. B. (2004). Fast food, race/ethnicity, and income. *American Journal of Preventive Medicine*, *27,* 211-217.

Bodor, J. N., Rose, D., Farley, T. A., Swalm, C. & Scott, S. K. (2008). Neighborhood fruit and vegetable availability and consumption: The role of small food stores in an urban environment. *Public Health Nutrition*, *11(4)*, 413-420.

Bowman, S. A., Gortmaker, S. L., Ebbeling, C. B., Pereira, M. A. & Ludwig, D. S. (2004). Effects of fast-food consumption on energy intake and diet quality among children in a national household survey. *Pediatrics*, *113*, 112-118.

Centers for Disease Control and Prevention, National Center for Health Statistics. (2006). *Prevalence of overweight among children and adolescents: United States, 2003-2004.* Retrieved June 10, 2008, from http://www.cdc.gov/nchs/products/pubs/pubd/hestats/overweight/overwght_child_03.htm

Cutler, D. M., Glaeser, E. L. & Shapiro, J. M. (2003). Why have Americans become more obese? *The Journal of Economic Perspectives*, *17(3)*, 93-118.

Darmon, N. & Drewnowski, A. (2008). Does social class predict diet quality? *American Journal of Clinical Nutrition*, *87(5)*, 1107-1117.

Food Marketing Institute. (2006). *U.S. grocery shopper trends 2006*. Arlington, VA: Author.

Glanz, K., Sallis, J., Saelens, B. E. & Frank, L. D. (2007). Nutrition environment measures survey in stores (NEMS-S): Development and evaluation. *American Journal of Preventive Medicine*, *32*, 282-289.

Glanz, K., Resnicow, K., Seymour, J., Hoy, K., Stewart, H., Lyons, M., et al. (2007). How major restaurant chains plan their menus: The role of profit, demand, and health. *American Journal of Preventive Medicine*, *32*, 383-3 88.

Golan, M. & Crow, S. (2004). Targeting parents exclusively in the treatment of childhood obesity: Long-term results. *Obesity Reviews*, *12*, 357-361.

Golan, M., Weizman, A., Apter, A. & Fainaru, M. (1998). Parents as the exclusive agents of change in the treatment of childhood obesity. *The American Journal of Clinical Nutrition*, *67*, 1130-1135.

Guthrie, J. F., Lin, B. H. & Frazao, E. (2002). Role of food prepared away from home in the American diet, 1977-1978 vs. 1994-1996: Changes and consequences. *Journal of Nutrition and Health Behavior*, *34*, 140-150.

Horowitz, C. R., Colson, K. A., Hebert, P. L. & Lancaster, K. (2004). Barriers to buying healthy foods for people with diabetes: Evidence of environmental disparities. *American Journal of Public Health*, *94(9)*, 1549-1554.

Institute of Medicine. (2004). *Preventing childhood obesity: Health in the balance.* Washington, DC: Author.

Kolodinsky, J. & Cranwell, M. (2000). The poor pay more? Now they don't even have a store to choose from: Bringing a supermarket back to the city. *Consumer Interests Annual*, *46*, 24-29.

J. P., Koplan, C. T. Liverman, & V. I. Kraak, (Eds.). (2005). *Preventing childhood obesity: Health in the balance.* Washington, DC: National Academies Press.

Larson, N., Story, M. & Nelson, M. C. (2008). Restaurant realities: Inequalities in access to healthy restaurant choices. In *Healthy eating research: A research brief.* Princeton, NJ: Robert Wood Johnson Foundation. Retrieved November 10, 2008, from http://www.healthyeatingresearch.org/uploads/COBbriefrestaurant2008.pdf

Lewis, L. B., Sloane, D. C., Nascimento, L. M., Diamant, A. L., Guinyard, J. J., Yancey, A. K., et al. (2005). African Americans' access to healthy food options in south Los Angeles restaurants. *American Journal of Public Health*, *95*, 668-673.

MacCrory, M. A., Fuss, P. J., Hays, H. P., Vinken, A. G., Greenberg, A. S. & Roberts, S. B. (1999). Overeating in America: Association between restaurant food consumption and body fatness in healthy adult men and women ages 19-80. *Obesity Research*, *7*, 564-571.

Miech, R. A., Kumanyika, S. K., Stettler, N., Link, B. G., Phelan, J. C. & Chang, V. W. (2006). Trends in the association of poverty with overweight among U.S. adolescents, 1971-2004. *Journal of the American Medical Association*, *295(20)*, 23 85-2393.

Mikkelsen, L. & Chehimi, S. (2007). *The links between the neighborhood food environment and childhood nutrition*. Princeton, NJ: Robert Wood Johnson Foundation. Retrieved August 5, 2009, from www.rwjf.org/pdf/foodenvironment

Moore, L. V. & Diez Roux, A. V. (2006). Associations of neighborhood characteristics with the location and type of food stores. *American Journal of Public Health*, *96(2)*, 325-331.

Morland, K., Wing, S. & Diez Roux, A. (2002). The contextual effect of the local food environment on residents' diets: The atherosclerosis risk in communities study. *American Journal of Public Health*, *92(11)*, 1761-1767.

Morland, K., Wing, S., Diez Roux, A. & Poole, C. (2002). Neighborhood characteristics associated with the location of food stores and food services places. *American Journal of Preventive Medicine*, *22*, 23-29.

Newby, P. K. (2007). Are dietary intakes and eating behaviors related to childhood obesity? A comprehensive review of the evidence. *Journal of Law, Medicine & Ethics*, *35(1)*, 3 5-60.

Ogden, C. L., Carroll, M. D. & Flegal, K. M. (2008). High body mass index for age among U.S. children and adolescents, 2003-2006. *Journal of the American Medical Association*, *299(20)*, 2401-2405.

Ogden, C. L., Carroll, M. D., Curtin, L. R., McDowell, M. A., Tabak, C. J. & Flegal, K. M. (2006). Prevalence of overweight and obesity in the United States, 1999-2004. *Journal of the American Medical Association*, *295*, 1549-1555.

Ohri-Vachaspati, P. & Leviton, L. C. (in press). Measuring food environments: A guide to available instruments. *American Journal of Health Promotion*.

Patton, M. Q. (1997). *Utilization-focused evaluation: The new century text.* Thousand Oaks, CA: Sage Publications.

Patton, M. Q. (2002). *Qualitative research methods & evaluation methods.* Thousand Oaks, CA: Sage Publications.

Pereira, M. A., Kartashov, A. I., Ebbeling, C. B., Van Horn, L., Slattery, M. L., Jacobs, D. R., Jr., et al. (2005). Fast-food habits, weight gain, and insulin resistance (the CARDIA study): 15-year prospective analysis. *Lancet*, *365*, 36-42.

Powell, L. M., Slater, S., Mirtcheva, D., Bao, Y. & Chaloupka, F. J. (2007). Food store availability and neighborhood characteristics in the United States. *Preventive Medicine*, *44*, 189-195.

Sallis, J. F. & Glanz, K. (2006). The role of built environments in physical activity, eating, and obesity in childhood. *The Future of Children*, *16(1)*, 89-108.

Schwartz, M. B. & Brownell, K. D. (2007). Actions necessary to prevent childhood obesity: Creating the climate for change. *Journal of Law, Medicine & Ethics*, *35(1)*, 78-89.

Swinburn, B. A., Metcalf, P. A. & Ley, S. J. (2001). Long-term (5-year) effects of a reduced-fat diet intervention in individuals with glucose intolerance. *Diabetes Care*, *24*, 619-624.

Taubes, G. (1997). New study says low-fat diet can lower blood pressure. *Science*, *276(5311)*, 350.

Thomson, O., Ballew, C., Resnicow, K., Must, A., Bardini, L. G., Cyn, H., et al. (2004). Food purchased away from home as a predictor of change in BMI Z-score among girls. *International Journal of Obesity*, *28*, 282-289.

Turrell, G., Hewitt, B., Patterson, C. & Oldenburg, B. (2003). Measuring socioeconomic position in dietary research: Is choice of socio-economic indicator important? *Public Health Nutrition*, *6*, 191-201.

U.S. Department of Agriculture, Agricultural Marketing Service. (2007). *Wholesale and farmers markets.* Retrieved June 10, 2008, from http://www.ams.usda.gov/AMSv1.0/ams.fetchTemplateData.do?template=TemplateA&navID=WholesaleandFarmersMarkets&leftNav=WholesaleandFarmersMarkets&page=WholesaleAndFarmersMarkets&acct=AMSPW

Wang, Y. & Beydoun, M. A. (2007). The obesity epidemic in the United States—Gender, age, socioeconomic, racial/ethnic, and geographic characteristics: A systematic review and meta- regression analysis. *Epidemiologic Reviews*, *29*, 6-28.

Wang, M. C., Kim, S., Gonzalez, A. A., MacLeod, K. E. & Winkleby, M. A. (2007). Socioeconomic and food-related physical characteristics of the neighborhood environment are associated with body mass index. *Journal of Epidemiology and Community Health*, *61(6)*, 491-498.

Wholey, J. S. (2004). Evaluability assessment. In J. S., Wholey, H. P. Hatry, & K. E. Newcomer, (Eds.), *Handbook of practical program evaluation*, (33-62). San Francisco, CA: Jossey-Bass.

In: Prevention of Childhood Obesity ISBN: 978-1-61209-962-0
Editor: Christina V. Mancuso, pp. 101-137

Chapter 3

LOCAL WELLNESS POLICY

Christina V. Mancuso

ACKNOWLEDGMENTS

This project is a collaborative effort led by a team from the Robert Wood Johnson Foundation (RWJF); the Centers for Disease Control and Prevention's (CDC) Division of Nutrition, Physical Activity and Obesity; Division of Adolescent and School Health; and Division of Adult and Community Health's Prevention Research Centers Program Office; and the CDC Foundation. The project team is advised by the Funder's Advisory Committee, which includes representatives from the RWJF, the National Institutes of Health, the U.S. Department of Agriculture (USDA), WK Kellogg Foundation, and Kaiser Permanente. ICF Macro, an ICF International Company, serves as the coordinating center for the project.

We are grateful to the staff at numerous schools for welcoming members of our project team to their sites and allowing us to learn more about their exemplary efforts. It is evident that there is a lot of energy and enthusiasm in the schools as it relates to the implementation of the local wellness policy. We applaud the tremendous efforts that schools have put forth in promoting health and wellness among students and staff.

I. Introduction

Background

Early Assessment of Programs and Policies to Prevent Childhood Obesity is a 2-year project to identify and assess local-level programs and policies that have been implemented with apparent success to prevent obesity by improving the eating habits and physical activity levels of children aged 3 to 17 years. In each year of the project, a systematic search process identified programs and policies, and then an expert panel suggested further exploration of the most promising programs and policies. Priority was given to programs and policies that addressed low-income populations and ethnic groups with disproportionate childhood obesity.

Purpose of Early Assessment

As the search for answers to effectively address childhood obesity continues, organizations and communities across the country are experimenting with various strategies aimed at changing children's environments to prevent obesity. The early assessment model is a process to screen environmental interventions for those that promise to be most effective in preventing childhood obesity, but lack empirical evidence about their effectiveness. Identifying these most promising projects could potentially lead to more rigorous evaluations in the future.

As part of the early assessment process, the evaluability method was used to assess the plausibility and feasibility of selected programs and policies that were identified as promising during the search process and selected by the expert panel. Evaluability assessment is a process in which evaluators work with program administrators and stakeholders to determine an initiative's readiness for evaluation (Patton, 1997). It involves clarifying goals and program design by specifying the program model, determining stakeholders' views on the important issues, and exploring program reality (Wholey, 2004). Evaluability assessments can help determine whether a rigorous evaluation study (e.g., an experimental evaluation such as a randomized control trial) is feasible and merited for a particular program or policy. As such, they can help avoid premature investment in rigorous evaluation of programs or policies that have not been adequately implemented and allow evaluation resources to be targeted to programs or policies deemed ready for rigorous evaluation.

Focus Areas

During the first year of the project, the Funder's Advisory Committee identified three thematic areas: child care programs and policies in afterschool and day care settings, programs or policies increasing access to healthier foods, and local wellness policies (LWPs). Synthesis reports have been prepared for each of these thematic areas.

This synthesis report focuses on the evaluability assessments conducted on LWPs. It describes the extent to which LWPs have been implemented and the limitations of implementation in six school districts across the nation. The report concludes with lessons learned and recommendations to inform future implementation by district and school personnel and other key decision makers.

Relevant Literature

Among children aged 6 to 11 years, 33.3% are overweight or obese; among adolescents aged 12 to 19 years, 34.1% are overweight or obese (Ogden, Carroll, & Flegal, 2008). With approximately 55 million children and adolescents enrolled in schools (grades K to 12), schools can play a critical role in influencing health, particularly healthy eating and physical activity, among children and adolescents (U.S. Census Bureau, 2006; Wechsler, McKenna, Lee, & Deitz, 2004).

In recognition of the role that schools play in improving health and in response to the growing obesity epidemic, Congress passed the Child Nutrition and Women, Infants, and Children (WIC) Reauthorization Act of 2004, which required each school district participating in a federally funded meal program to establish a local wellness policy (LWP). The LWP should include nutrition guidelines for all foods and beverages available on school campuses during the school day; set goals for nutrition education, physical activity, and other school-based activities designed to promote student wellness; and describe how implementation of the policy will be monitored. School districts were also required to involve parents, students, the local school food authority, the school board, and school administrators in the development of the policy. School districts were expected to adopt the policy by August 2006 and were encouraged to implement the policy. Technical assistance for policy development, implementation, and evaluation was provided by federal agencies (Department of Health and Human Services and the Department of Education) to states that, in turn, provided technical assistance to school districts. A number of national organizations also provided technical assistance, such as Action for Healthy Kids and the School Nutrition Association.

Research suggests that school health programs can promote healthy eating and physical activity among children and adolescents; however, limited data exist as to the impact of policies on these behaviors (Centers for Disease Control and Prevention, 1996, 1997; Gortmaker et al., 1999; Hoelscher et al., 2004). A recent study to assess school health policies and programs found that only 17.0% of districts required that schools make beverages meeting specific nutritional standards, such as bottled water or low-fat milk, available to students. In addition, only 6.6% of district policies required that schools make fruits and vegetables available to students whenever food was offered or sold (O'Toole, Anderson, Miller, & Guthrie, 2007). When physical activity was examined, only 67.8% of elementary schools provided daily recess for students in all grades (Lee, Burgeson, Fulton, & Spain, 2007). As demonstrated by these data, before the law requiring LWPs, districts and schools had very few policies and practices in place that promoted healthy eating and physical activity. As a result, it is important to understand the extent to which LWPs have been implemented and the implications for school health.

II. Methods

Nomination of Programs and Policies

The project team solicited nominations for LWPs between March and May 2007 from school districts across the United States through postings on a variety of listservs (e.g., the Comprehensive Health Education Network) and through direct contact with the Centers for Disease Control and Prevention's (CDC) Division of Adolescent and School Health project officers and funded school health program coordinators. Nominated policies were eligible for inclusion in the project if they were adopted by a school district; implemented in multiple district schools during the 2006–2007 school year; included all of the required components of the wellness policy; had not been previously evaluated; and had been monitored over a period of time. Policies that met our inclusion criteria were examined further based on the content and quality of the written policy using specific criteria (see Appendix A for a list of criteria) that addressed the use of evidence-based methods for promoting behavior change. For example, one criterion stated, "Physical education is offered daily (i.e., 150 minutes per week at the elementary school level, 225 minutes per week at the high school level)." Each criterion received a score of 1 point if the criterion was addressed in the policy or 0 points if the criterion was not addressed in the policy. The scores for each policy were totaled, then policies were rank ordered based on the scores. The highest-scoring policies (ranging from 0 to 49 points) were reviewed by the expert panel. A total of 146 policies were nominated, 58 met our criteria for inclusion, and the 25 highest-scoring policies were reviewed by the expert panel.

Criteria and Selection of Policies for Evaluability Assessments

We convened a panel of 15 experts in evaluation, measurement, nutrition, physical activity, school- aged youth, and community programs in March 2007. Specific criteria to select policies for evaluability assessment were developed by the project team in collaboration with the expert panel. These criteria included potential impact of the policy; innovativeness; reach to target population; acceptability to stakeholders; feasibility of implementation; feasibility of adoption; sustainability; generalizability; and staff and organizational capacity of the implementers (see Appendix B for a detailed description of each criterion). The expert panel reviewed prepared summaries of each of the 25 highest-scoring local wellness policies, scored each policy on each criterion through an Internet-based survey tool, and made recommendations on which policies would receive evaluability assessments. After each panel member scored each policy and discussed each policy as a group, six LWPs were recommended for evaluability assessments.

Local Wellness Policy Evaluability Assessment Site Visit

Each evaluability assessment involved (1) a review of background documentation about the program or policy; (2) the development of a program or policy logic model to outline program goals and activities; and (3) a 2.5-day site visit, in which trained site visitors assessed implementation, data collection, and evaluation capacity through interviews with program staff and partners. One district per state was visited in Arizona, Minnesota, New Mexico, and Texas and two districts were visited in Wyoming. Each evaluability assessment site visit was conducted by two site visitors who traveled to the school districts. Interviews were conducted with individuals involved with the policy, such as school district personnel, principals, teachers, parents, community partners, and other stakeholders. Interview questions addressed policy development, implementation, evaluation, and funding (see Appendix C for the list of questions). The project team and expert panel reviewed the findings from all the evaluability assessments to determine the degree of promise of the programs and policies and their readiness for rigorous evaluation.

Data Analysis

Site visit reports were created from each site visit and were the primary data sources for this synthesis report. Reports were analyzed for themes using open coding of qualitative data (Bernard, 2000). Three team members initially identified codes in the texts of the site visit reports. Each individual developed codes independently after reviewing the site visit reports, then compared and discussed similarities and differences to arrive at a single comprehensive list of codes for analysis (Patton, 2002). One team member then coded all reports from each site. ATLAS.ti (version 5.0) was used to categorize and sort data within codes. Secondary data sources included expert panel preliminary review perspectives and expert panel postsite visit recommendations. Site visitors have reviewed a draft of the results section of this report for accuracy of interpretation.

III. Background

District Characteristics

School district enrollment ranged from 2,600 students across 10 schools to 41,444 students across 66 schools. Although the majority of students in three of the school districts were white, the other three districts were more racially and ethnically diverse. In two school districts, approximately 50% of the student body was Hispanic and in a third district 60% of the students were Asian American or African American. Four of the six school districts were in urban areas. Among the six school districts, 16% to 70% of students were eligible for free and reduced-price lunches (see Table 1).

Other Health-Related Policies

Three districts had previous experience with school health and wellness at the district level before the 2004 Child Nutrition and WIC Reauthorization Act. In 2002, two school districts participated in the Urban School Health Leadership Institute that facilitated the development of an interdisciplinary wellness leadership team for each school district. The institute was sponsored by the American Cancer Society and CDC to help school districts develop a systematic and coordinated approach to addressing health and safety issues that interfere with student success. The third district had a physical education faculty member who was the dedicated lead for physical education and school health initiatives in the district before the mandate.

However, with the exception of LWPs, districts had few policies that addressed student health and wellness. One district had a policy that addressed each component of a coordinated school health program as mandated by the state education agency. Four other districts had at least one policy that addressed one or more of the following: school nutrition services management, the free and reduced-price lunch program, prohibition of foods that did not meet specific nutritional standards from being sold in school nutrition services areas, graduation requirements for physical education, and the creation of healthy and safe environments. Only one district had a policy that addressed what foods and beverages could be brought into the school by students and parents.

Development of the LWPs

All six school districts intensively involved key stakeholders in the policy development process. In general, LWPs were developed by small teams of individuals (i.e., writing teams) representing school districts (e.g., assistant superintendent, director of student services, director of school nutrition services, director of health services), schools (e.g., principals, teachers, parents, and students), and communities (e.g., local health department representatives, community-based organizations). Writing teams were often a subcommittee of the districtwide school health advisory council or wellness committee, although in one district the writing team included three district-level administrators (the school nutrition services director and assistant director, and the director of curriculum), who presented the policy to the school health advisory council for review. Wellness committees were most commonly led by school nutrition services staff at the district level. Although the composition of wellness teams varied, they were most likely to include district-level school nutrition and student health services representatives, dietitians, principals, school board members, health and physical education teachers, parents, and community members (representing the medical community, public health department, and university).

All LWPs were developed after a review of resources, including Federal and State nutrition guidelines, national and State physical education standards, and sample policies from State and national organizations. State Action for Healthy Kids documents were also a common resource for policy development.

Two school districts used the coordinated school health program (Joint Committee on Health Education and Promotion Terminology, 2001) and the learner support framework (Adelman & Taylor, 2005) to develop their policy. The learner support framework shifts resource teams in middle schools from a focus on case management to a broader focus on the environment.

Goals and Outcomes of the LWPs

The six LWPs included goals that varied in content and degree of specificity. Most goals were consistent with the required nutrition and physical activity components of the LWP. The goals addressed the provision of nutritious meals and snacks, nutrition education, opportunities to increase physical activity, and the creation of healthy school environments. Policies also addressed instilling lifelong healthy behaviors related to healthy eating and physical activity. For example, a common nutrition education goal was that each school would offer a sequential, interdisciplinary, comprehensive standards-based curriculum designed to provide students with the knowledge and skills necessary to promote healthy and enjoyable eating habits that last a lifetime. Four of the six policies were prescriptive, outlining in detail how goals were to be achieved. These policies generally used strong language such as "will offer" and "shall offer." The two less prescriptive policies either recommended activities that could be implemented to achieve goals or indicated that schools "will strive" to meet specified goals.

All six LWPs stated that nutrition guidelines for reimbursable school meals would be at least as restrictive as the *Dietary Guidelines for Americans* established by the U.S. Department of Agriculture (USDA) and the Department of Health and Human Services. In addition, three school districts specified adherence to State-level nutrition standards for reimbursable meals in their policies.

Each school district outlined in varying degrees of specificity, guidelines for foods and beverages available on school campuses outside of the school meal program (i.e., competitive foods) (Institute of Medicine, 2007). Five of the six policies referenced national nutrition guidance (i.e., *U.S. Dietary Guidelines*) as the basis for the district's nutrition guidelines for competitive foods. Two districts also referenced State nutrition standards as the basis for the district's nutrition guidelines for competitive foods. All six LWPs (whether included in the policy or as an additional document) provided some guidance about the types of foods and beverages that should be offered to, or restricted from, students. This guidance ranged from lists of suggested food and beverage items to detailed lists of foods and beverages with specified portion sizes, calorie count, fat content, and/or comparisons of good and better food and beverage choices. For example, one district's policy specified the following: all foods and beverages in each school must meet the district standards for foods and beverages; choices will not exceed 2.5 servings; single-serving-size snacks should have no more than 6 grams of fat; milk, water, 100% juice, and sports drinks are allowed; and only fruits, dried fruits, and vegetables prepared/packaged without added fat, sugar, sodium, or coatings other than those used for food preservation are allowed.

Less commonly noted were standards for physical activity or physical education. Only one school district referenced national physical education standards for its policy guidance.

Staff developed logic models that describe many of the expected outcomes of the policy implementation (see Appendix D for a sample logic model). In general, short-term (1–3 years) outcomes included full implementation of the LWP; increased availability of healthier food and beverage options in schools; more alternative or healthier fundraising events, parties, or snack options; and increased parent and community awareness and involvement. Less common were short-term outcomes for increasing professional development, opportunities for physical activity, and staff wellness. Intermediate (3–5 years) outcomes included increased consumption of healthier foods and beverages, increased academic scores, and increased physical activity among students. Although less commonly noted on the logic models, long-term (4–6 years) outcomes focused mainly on measured improvements in weight status as measured by body mass index (BMI).

Across all six districts, stakeholders agreed on the goals, activities, and outcomes of their LWP. Each district identified some level of initial opposition to the policy from stakeholders (e.g., parents, students, and school personnel), which had since been largely overcome. When interviewed, stakeholders discussed the logic model created by the project staff for their school district. Stakeholders were positive and agreed with the logic model components (inputs, activities, outputs, and outcomes).

Each district's policy was expected to include a plan for measuring implementation, including designating one or more persons within the district or at each school charged with operational responsibility for ensuring that each school fulfilled the district's LWP. In general, local wellness policies identified either the superintendent or members of the school health advisory councils as having oversight of implementation. Local wellness policies included an annual report component describing the policy's implementation to school boards. Local wellness policies for all six districts lacked detailed descriptions on how monitoring and evaluation would be conducted.

Target Audiences

The primary target audience for all six LWPs was all students in the district enrolled in grades K to 12. Three school districts also identified district- and school-level staff, parents, and community members as part of their target audience.

IV. Logic Model

As part of the evaluability assessments, each district developed a logic model describing inputs and activities and outputs. An example of a logic model can be found in Appendix D. The next two sections describe (a) inputs and (b) activities and outputs from each of the six districts.

Inputs

Funding

Districts receive few or no resources for the full implementation of LWPs. Despite this lack of direct funding, districts have been able to use a combination of Federal funds, State funds, district funds, and funding from local organizations to implement various aspects of LWPs. In the six districts, financial support for implementing the LWP primarily included Federal funding (e.g., Title I funds, Carol M. White Physical Education Program [PEP] grants). In one district, the State legislature appropriated $115,199 to cover the costs of providing free breakfast for all students in seven elementary schools. Another district was able to appropriate $57,500 of district funds for implementation. Funds were used to offset the revenue losses from vending machine changes, support a wellness coordinator position, support healthy school projects, and supplement nutritional provisions for school lunches and snacks. Two other school districts appropriated funds (up to $10,000 in one district and up to $30,000 in the other) to offset the projected loss in revenue that might have resulted from implementation of nutrition guidelines in the first year. Other sources of financial support came from local grants from companies and organizations (e.g., city council, State department of education).

In at least five of the six districts, school nutrition services absorbed much of the costs for implementing the LWP. The operating structure of school nutrition services varied from district to district, with some operating as nonprofits. As a result, it was essential that these entities not create a deficit due to increased costs of offering healthy foods. School nutrition services personnel across the districts agreed that serving more fruits and vegetables increased costs. One school district estimated a 1.5% increase in food and beverage purchasing costs, adjusted for inflation, due to changes resulting from the LWP. Some school nutrition directors reported offering the least expensive fruits and vegetables, and using some canned fruits and vegetables to keep costs down. One district increased the price of school lunch by 10 cents. In another district, school nutrition services funded the school health coordinator position, in part, with assistance from revenues supplied by Medicaid from student health services. School nutrition services also assumed costs related to printing, materials, and other resources to support the policy.

The financial impact of the change of vending options varied across school districts. For example, in one district, although $30,000 was appropriated to cover vending machine revenue loss, only one school in the district reported a loss (of $1,500). Another school district reported a 73% loss in commissions paid to schools for a 2-month period during the first year of policy implementation.

Funding for physical education was particularly difficult. Only two of the six districts were able to garner additional funding to hire more physical education teachers for the upcoming 2008–2009 school year.

Staffing

Of the six school districts, three had individuals at the district level dedicated to overseeing the implementation of the LWP, and two were affiliated with the school nutrition services department. These individuals had a strong presence in the schools in day-to-day policy management and made a significant impact on schools in achieving their goals. One reported to both the director of school nutrition services and the director of health services. In another district, a registered dietitian was hired.

District-level staff committed to implementing the LWP was critical. One district lost its district- level LWP champion to a new position. As the director of student services, this person headed the wellness program directly under the superintendent, and supervised the school nurses, physical education and health education teachers, and guidance counselors. The district decided not to fill this position and reorganized the program so the components were less integrated organizationally; no one directly reported to the superintendent. This was a great loss for the district and weakened the district's implementation of the LWP.

LWP implementation in all six districts benefited from having identified contacts at the school level or local champions. Four of the six school districts had school-level liaisons for the LWP. These liaisons included individuals (e.g., teachers and nurses) or small teams in schools that communicated with district-level personnel regarding the LWP or activities related to it.

School districts in this study partnered with other district-level entities and organizations and universities which facilitated the policy implementation because of the extra manpower the partnerships provided. Several district-level partnerships were identified, including the curriculum and instruction department, office of fund development (grant writing), and the business office. Partnerships with universities typically facilitated nutrition education and professional development for physical education instructors. Other partners included local public health departments and municipal departments of parks and recreation, whereby resources for nutrition education and physical activity could be leveraged.

Activities and Outputs

None of the six local wellness policies was fully implemented. At the time of the evaluability assessment site visits, school districts and schools had just begun the second year of implementation. Participating school districts had made significant progress in implementing nutrition goals, but less progress in implementing physical activity goals.

Vending

The six districts had made great progress in implementing nutrition guidelines for vending machines. In two districts, vending was limited before the congressional mandate. In one district, soda was eliminated from vending machines in all schools in 2003. In the other district, there was never food vending at the elementary school level. In the two districts in which the vending contract was centralized at the district level, progress was quite visible. These districts, for the most part, had vending machines that were stocked with food and beverage options meeting nutritional standards.

During the first implementation year in one district, snack and beverage options meeting nutritional standards (e.g., water, flavored water, energy drinks, milk products, or juices) were phased into the vending machines in 50% of schools. By October of the following school year, all vending machines in the district offered snack and beverage options meeting nutritional standards. In addition, all vending machines were on timers during the school day, which allowed limited opportunity for vending purchases. In this school district, vendors voluntarily offered more snack and beverage alternatives (at least 15 different alternatives) that met nutritional standards. However, vending machines in employee lounges at some schools still carried beverage options not meeting nutritional standards—sending a mixed message to students.

School Nutrition Services

A strong emphasis was placed on improving food quality for school meals across all six districts, from offering whole grains and reduced-fat dairy products to offering more baked foods and foods with reduced sodium. In one district, ensuring healthy, appealing, and culturally appropriate offerings was a top priority. The school district worked with a professional chef to improve its recipes, and also prepared ethnic foods. The district made an effort to identify the preferences of the students and to meet them (e.g., cutting apples and oranges because students prefer them that way). This district had a centralized nutrition service that prepared the food for all schools in the school district, which enabled them to standardize and control the food available districtwide. Another district placed health bars in schools. Health bars are buffet-style carts that offer a variety of fresh fruits and vegetables daily. Two health bars were placed in each of its 26 elementary schools, and several health bars were available at the secondary level as well. A third district promoted breakfast in the classroom, offering free, healthy breakfast for elementary school students in morning classes, instead of in the cafeteria. This program was implemented in half of the elementary schools in the district. Two districts were in the process of implementing (or had already implemented) USDA's Healthier US Challenge criteria in elementary schools and were working on expanding the guidelines to all schools. However, a variety of challenges remained with regard to nutrition in schools. For example, students did not have enough time to eat lunch according to staff. In addition, there was limited control at the school level to choose the foods they served, and increased costs were associated with serving more fruits and vegetables.

Fundraising and Special Events

The six school districts were struggling to conduct fundraising using foods that met nutritional standards or nonfood items. Many of the LWPs discouraged, but did not prohibit, teacher use of food as a reward and parent-supplied food for parties. One district limited classes to one birthday celebration per month, while another specified two events per year where foods not meeting nutritional standards could be served (e.g., cake). Across all districts there had been some degree of resistance from teachers, parents, and students regarding restrictions on fundraising and food for classroom celebrations.

Two districts had systems in place to monitor the foods and beverages used for fundraising activities and school-sponsored events. One district partnered with the district's business office, which reviewed the purchase orders, to ensure food options that met nutritional standards were available for students at school events or fundraisers. Purchase orders requesting foods and beverages for an event had to specify at least 50% of food and beverage options meeting nutritional standards. In addition, those interested in holding a fundraiser were required to participate in a training about the LWP and sign a memorandum of understanding regarding the LWP.

Nutrition Education

The provision of nutrition education across all grade levels was a challenge for the school districts. In general, nutrition education was not regularly or consistently offered to K to 12 students, and some of the staff who provided nutrition education lacked the necessary training.

Four of the six school districts identified a nutrition education or health education curriculum (including nutrition) that was being implemented. The two remaining school districts were either trying to identify a curriculum or had no nutrition or health education curriculum. For example, for the past 7 years the evidence-based Coordinated Approach to Child Health (CATCH) program was implemented in all elementary schools in one school district (Perry et al., 1990). The program integrates nutrition policy and education with physical education policy and curriculum.

The degree of implementation of nutrition education varied by district, and even more so by schools within the district. Across all districts, implementation of nutrition education was heavily targeted at the elementary school level and generally did not exist at the secondary level. Furthermore, only a fraction of schools in school districts that identified a nutrition education or health education curriculum actually offered nutrition education consistently. For example, in one school district only 14 of the 24 elementary schools offered nutrition education using a standard nutrition education curriculum and even then instruction occurred only once a month. In another district, nutrition education was provided on an as-requested basis. Teachers, however, were encouraged by school districts to integrate nutrition education into core subjects.

The National Health Education Standards (Joint Committee on National Health Education Standards, 2007) recommends that nutrition education be provided within a comprehensive health education curriculum and taught by trained teachers; however, only a small proportion of teachers in the districts that provided nutrition education were trained. Nutrition education teachers were most likely to receive training when the curriculum was first adopted, but refresher courses were less likely to be offered. Furthermore, new teachers who were not trained when the curriculum was initially adopted generally did not receive training on the nutrition education curriculum. In districts where teachers were encouraged to integrate nutrition education into core subjects such as math and science, many lacked the nutritional knowledge necessary for proper instruction. District and school personnel cited limited funding, competing demands for time, State requirements for a strong emphasis on academic instruction, and national and State testing as the primary reasons for the lack of nutrition education instruction and training.

Physical Education

In general, limited physical education was offered and limited opportunities for physical activity were available across all grade levels. In all six school districts, there was growing momentum for increasing the number of certified physical education teachers.

According to the National Association for Sport & Physical Education, the national recommendation for physical education is a minimum of 150 minutes per week at the elementary school level and 225 minutes per week at the middle and high school levels (National Association for Sport & Physical Education, 2005). Few of the districts and schools met this recommendation. In one school district, health and physical education time were combined at the elementary and middle school levels (90 minutes at the elementary school level and 200 minutes at the middle school level), making it difficult to determine how much physical education was being provided. At the high school level, one credit (two semesters) of physical education was required for graduation. At another school district, elementary school students received 40 minutes of physical education once a week.

Although encouraged, before-, during-, and after-school physical activity remains a challenge to implement. Recess was available daily at the elementary school level in all six school districts and ranged from 20 to 40 minutes daily for elementary school students. Most LWPs encouraged schools to not remove recess opportunities as punishment and it was apparent that most schools were complying. Two districts provided districtwide in-service trainings on movement in the classroom (e.g., brain-based movement, Total Physical Response, Energizers). Many individual schools had after-school programs; however, programs focused on providing academic support with little opportunity for physical activity or lacked participation from students.

Participating district and school personnel cited many reasons for lack of a stronger emphasis on physical education, including weak State standards for physical education, limited budgets, competing demands for time, State requirements for a strong emphasis on other academic instruction, national and State testing, few physical education teachers, and poor scheduling. Furthermore, for many districts physical education was not centralized at the district level, and as a result the provision of physical education was left to the discretion of the school principal. For one district, the lack of progress was because of the lack of district-level staff responsible for physical education.

Other School-Based Activities

One common school-based activity that many of the six LWPs included was employee wellness promotion. Two districts made a concerted effort to promote employee wellness, with district-level support through a centralized health insurer. Health promotion activities across the two districts ranged from organized walking groups to health-related e-mail announcements regarding health assessments. Few schools in the remaining four school districts promoted employee wellness through activities such as walking groups, weight loss competitions, and by making student workout areas and equipment available to employees before and after school.

One district used healthy school plans (HSPs) to achieve policy goals at the school level. Each school was expected to submit two HSPs each school year that included activities addressing an LWP component (e.g., physical activity, nutrition, and education opportunities). In this district, funding was allocated for incentives for schools to carry out their HSPs. HSP activities ranged from creating a physical activity club to monthly label-reading sessions for students.

To encourage better nutritional intake among elementary school students in another school district, Recess Before Lunch (RBL) was promoted. As research suggests, RBL reduces classroom behavior issues and increases lunch consumption (Bergman, Buergel, Englund, & Femrite, 2004; Getlinger, Laughlin,

Bell, Akre, & Arjmandi, 1996). Approximately half of the elementary schools in the school district implemented this program.

V. Evaluation Activities

Evaluation was not the primary responsibility of district and school personnel implementing the LWP and, as such, many of the six school districts had only a modest capacity to evaluate implementation of their LWP. Districts were seeking evaluation assistance from other district offices that focused on assessment or evaluation, or from evaluation consultants. Several districts identified partners for evaluation, such as the Alliance for a Healthier Generation or academic institutions.

LWP evaluation activities among the six school districts that were underway focused on single initiatives rather than on implementation of the LWP as a whole, and lacked regularity and coordination among the components of the policy in the schools. Two of the six districts reported using an assessment tool during the first year to determine what aspects of the policy were being used and how implementation was occurring. For example, one district translated the policy components and stipulations into an instrument with a three-way rating system for each ("in place/under development/not in place"). These tools were to be completed by school nurses and signed off by principals; however, it might have been more fruitful if the wellness policy team completed the tool rather than one individual.

All six school districts had data sources available that could be used to monitor aspects of their LWP including surveys on student health behavior and outcomes (e.g., the Youth Risk Behavior Survey), health and fitness assessments, student school meal participation rates, information about the nutritional content of school meals, competitive food sales summaries, measures of student BMI, and various training participation rates (including trainings on LWP, nutrition, and physical activity). These data sources, however, were not coordinated, compared analytically, or used to make improvements. Even in districts in which some process evaluation had taken place, little was done to use the data to inform program development or identify and provide technical assistance to help schools meet LWP goals.

VI. Discussion

Plausibility

The fundamental premise that has guided LWP development for many of the six school districts is that schools play a key role in promoting student health, and can prevent childhood obesity through proper nutrition and physical activity (Wechsler, McKenna, Lee, and Deitz, 2004). This foundation, along with using additional frameworks (e.g., learner support framework, coordinated school health approach) by two school districts in informing their policy, makes it plausible that LWP goals are achievable.

As a whole, the LWPs addressed the required components in a consistent and structured manner. The majority of the participating districts' policies used innovative approaches to address financial barriers to implementation (e.g., use of Title I funds, Carol M. White Physical Education Program [PEP] grants, and State and local organization funding).

It is plausible that full implementation of these LWPs will produce desired short-term outcomes. Specifically, achievable short-term outcomes include the availability of foods that meet nutritional standards during the school day and implementing physical activity opportunities at the elementary school level. In general, recess is offered daily, and physical education is available. Districts are making a concerted effort to meet the national physical education requirements despite barriers such as national and State standardized testing, which requires dedicated time for testing preparation, and shrinking budgets.

The LWPs can have a significant effect on the school environment of most students in these six school districts, with the extent of the impact varying given the different resources of each school district and school. The LWPs have increased awareness of the importance of healthy eating and physical activity among administrators, students, and parents. In addition, the availability of food and beverage options that meet nutritional standards has increased. In districts that serve a high proportion of free and reduced price school lunches, where students were more likely to consume breakfast and lunch at the school, the potential impact is even higher. Stronger community and parental support and involvement for carrying out the LWP are necessary for positive long-term outcomes.

Feasibility

It is feasible that various policy components will be used as designed, as districts strive for systematic, districtwide implementation. As described, for most school districts participating in this project, carrying out the LWP is ongoing and incremental. Schools with strong interest in implementation and strong leadership are more likely to have applied key components of the policy. Using districtwide curricula for nutrition, physical education, and oversight from a fully functioning school health advisory council are critical for full policy implementation.

Sustainability

Sustainability of various components of the LWPs is likely, despite the challenges experienced by the districts. Many schools have been successful in using low-cost strategies to implement LWPs.

However, many strategies rely on grant funding, which is less sustainable. Overall, sustainability is most likely achievable when aspects of the policy are implemented and controlled at the district level. In addition, sustainability is likely to occur when schools have the flexibility to tailor aspects of the policy to meet their needs. Sustainability is threatened when policy components rely on school-level implementation with district-level support, are not supported by State standards (e.g., physical education), and rely on external funding.

Generalizability to Similar Districts Implementing Local Wellness Policies

Various LWP components, programs, and strategies in these six districts are generalizable to other districts. The most generalizable component of the LWPs is the nutrition guidelines. Districts with centralized vending contracts are able to provide uniform availability of healthy food and beverage options through vending machines. General programs or curricula used in these six districts included Recess before Lunch, Breakfast in the Classroom, and Coordinated Approach to Child Health (CATCH). It is likely that these programs could be transferred to other settings and adopted for different populations because the programs target school environments that are locally controlled and potentially modifiable (e.g., the school schedule, determining which competitive foods may be served on campus).

VII. Key Lessons Learned

Key lessons were learned through the evaluability assessment site visits about the planning, implementation, and evaluation of the LWP's mandated by the 2004 Child Nutrition and WIC Reauthorization Act. For many of the school districts, this law supported initiatives that were under way to improve the healthy eating and physical activity behaviors of school-aged children. For other school districts, it provided impetus to take the necessary steps toward improving these behaviors among children and adolescents. As a result of the policy, there has been an increased awareness among stakeholders about the need to improve opportunities for healthy eating and physical activity for school-aged youth and the role schools can play in promoting a healthy school environment.

Stakeholders developed the policy and formed coalitions, advisory councils, and committees with a focus on school health. Not only were wellness issues discussed regarding the policy, but a framework was developed whereby other school health issues could be discussed (e.g., asthma and mental health), and an opportunity to link various other school health initiatives together was provided. Furthermore, a variety of partnerships were developed with other departments within the district and with outside agencies such as public health departments and universities.

Stakeholder involvement, although required for developing the LWP, was equally important for the policy implementation and sustainability. Since the development of the LWP, stakeholder involvement has waned, with a loss of momentum for implementation. In particular, parent and community involvement has not been sustained. Clear roles for stakeholder involvement in implementation and evaluation need to be identified and articulated, especially for community partners and parents. Identifying local-level champions will also keep the momentum going during implementation. For example, in some districts school-level champions (principals, teachers, and parents) played a key role by advocating for the LWP.

District-level coordination of LWP activities is beneficial for implementing the policy. LWP coordinators fostered positive relationships between district and school personnel. Their presence in schools also served to garner support for the policy, facilitate coordination of activities, and foster accurate communication about the policy to a variety of stakeholders.

Communication about the policy with the broader community is critical. In many districts, fear regarding the implementation of the LWP resulted from a lack of clear and consistent messages about it. Among school personnel, there was also fear regarding the loss of revenue due to vending changes. To an extent, teachers and principals believed that many parents were still unclear about what types of foods could be brought into schools. Plans for communicating with all stakeholders about the LWP need to be developed and implemented by school districts.

Several districts and schools benefitted from having a dedicated budget to support the implementation of their LWP. School districts require resources to fully implement the policy. In particular, financial support is needed for additional teachers, teacher training, and to cover increased costs related to offering healthier food items. Funding is also needed for in-service trainings on nutrition education and physical education among teachers. Many schools are struggling with implementing nutrition guidelines for fundraising and classroom foods. Schools lack sufficient resources to adequately implement healthy or nonfood item alternatives for fundraising. As a first step, school districts should strategically identify resources that can be used to facilitate the implementation of various components of the policy.

Districts and schools also need support from States in setting standards for health education and physical education. Without State standards on physical education, for example, students will not receive the amount and quality of physical education that is nationally recommended.

Although progress has been made in the implementation of LWPs, much of the work has occurred at the elementary school level. Districts described their target audience as being all grade levels; however, it is apparent that only certain aspects of the policy were reaching the entire student population. For example, in one school district the target audience had primarily been the elementary school level where more opportunities for nutrition education and physical activity had been provided. Standardized testing and accountability for academic subjects other than health and physical education have limited what schools make a priority at the secondary school level. Districts and schools should identify resources to assist with implementing nutrition education and physical activity goals, such as theory-based nutrition education curricula, resources to promote movement in the classroom, and standards-based physical education.

Table 1. District Characteristics.

School District	Number of Schools	Student Enrollment	Race/Ethnicity	Rural or Urban	Free/Reduced Price Lunch Rate	Plausibility	Feasibility	Potential Impact
A	10	2,600	White (84%) Black (<1.0%) Hispanic (11%) Asian/Pacific Islander (<1.0%) American Indian/Alaskan Native (<1.0%) Other (2%)	Rural	17%	It is plausible that nutrition knowledge will be increased.	Full implementation is supported by current infrastructure and could be enhanced with additional resources and school-based teams.	Potential impact is strongest at the elementary and middle school levels.
B	10	6,500	Hispanic (25%)	Rural	50%	It is plausible that desired outcomes will be achieved (to improve nutrition offerings and increase physical activity).	Feasibility could be enhanced by strengthening the district team and by increasing staff and resources for nutrition and physical education.	Potential impact is strongest at the elementary level and could be increased using a comprehensive community approach.
C	38	11,601	White (84%) Black (2%) Hispanic (6%) Other (2%)	Urban	33%	Plausibility is enhanced by the district's strong leadership and support, and development of tailored goals and objectives.	Feasibility is enhanced by the phased implementation of the policy and the dedicated funding.	There is the potential for significantly impacting the school environment;however, the extent of the impact would vary given the resources at individual schools.

School District	Number of Schools	Student Enrollment	Race/Ethnicity	Rural or Urban	Free/Reduced Price Lunch Rate	Plausibility	Feasibility	Potential Impact
D	20	14,000	White (31%) Black (24%) Hispanic (45%) American Indian (1%)	Urban	65%	Plausibility is increased by the use of evidence-based programs.	Feasibility is enhanced by the district's positive leadership and the conduct of yearly assessments.	The potential impact on the nutrition and physical activity environment is favorable.
E	35	23,000	White (25.6%) Black (2.4%) Hispanic (70.2%) Asian (1.0%) American Indian (0.8%)	Urban	53%	The use of scientifically sound nutritional programs increases plausibility.	Feasibility is strong for current programs.	Overall impact could be improved with the expansion of nutrition programs to upper grade levels and stronger physical education regulations.
F	66	41,444	White (26%) Black (30%) Hispanic (13%) American Indian (2%)	Urban	69%	Policy is guided by sound theoretical models. Plausibility is enhanced by a focus on the environment and cultural tailoring.	Feasibility is favorable due to central control of various components (e.g., nutrition services and vending).	Potential impact on nutrition (e.g. foods consumed by students) is high.

Districts and schools should consider using a systematic approach to implementing LWPs, such as the coordinated school health program. When the strengths and challenges of implementing the LWP are examined, they are consistent with the essential components of a coordinated school health program (coalitions, parent involvement, staff promotion, nutrition services, and physical education). Using the coordinated school health program model can help to address and coordinate the implementation of the LWP, while reducing the barriers to policy implementation.

Monitoring and evaluating the LWP is essential to determining how the policy is being used in schools. Many districts were not systematically monitoring their LWP. Without process evaluation data, it is difficult to get a clear picture of which schools are complying with all aspects of the policy and to identify areas in need of improvement. Districts need formal evaluation plans that clearly outline who will conduct the evaluation, what will be evaluated, what data sources will be used for the evaluation, how the evaluation will be conducted, and when the evaluation will occur. District school health advisory councils may need to use partnerships to take a more active role in monitoring and evaluating their LWPs.

VIII. Conclusion

The 2004 Child Nutrition and WIC Reauthorization Act has provided a strong platform for school health. Because most school districts across the nation are required by law to adopt LWPs, the importance and value of school health programs has been raised. LWPs serve as a catalyst, opportunity, and framework for needed change in schools to improve health. Many State agencies and school districts have recognized the need to improve their students' health by encouraging healthy eating and physical activity.

Among the six participating school districts, there have been a number of notable successes in implementing the policy. To date, LWPs have most influenced the nutrition environment through the availability of foods and beverages that meet nutritional standards to students at school. Other successes include improved quality of foods served to students, the availability of daily recess at the elementary school level, and increased support and promotion of employee wellness. Less progress has been made in the provision of nutrition education and in improving the physical activity behaviors of students.

Full implementation of the LWP is feasible, but not without accountability, State support, and funding. Without accountability, districts are not motivated to evaluate. A current barrier to monitoring and evaluation is weak policy language with no accountability mechanisms, no implementation checks, and no reporting. In addition, State support through adopting standards for health education and physical education, and the provision of technical assistance and necessary funding will give schools the tools needed to make nutrition and physical activity a priority.

This project has provided a unique opportunity to get a baseline understanding of school needs and to see what can actually be accomplished to promote health in schools through LWPs. Of the six LWPs that received an evaluability assessment, four have been deemed ready for evaluation. This is an exciting opportunity for us to begin to assess the impact of local wellness policies and look at the implications of this policy on school health.

APPENDIX A. LOCAL WELLNESS POLICY CRITERIA: CHECKLIST

Local Wellness Policy (LWP) Checklist

The LWP Checklist will be used to rank order local wellness policies, such that policies with higher scores will move on to be reviewed by the expert panel. Each criterion will receive a maximum score of 1 point (1 point if criterion is addressed in the policy or 0 points if the criterion is not addressed in the policy).

State:			**District Contact Name:**	
School District:			**Contact Information:**	
		Addressed in Policy	**Not Addressed in Policy**	**Note**
Nutrition Education				
	Nutrition education offered at all grade levels in the school.[1]			
	Topics of nutrition education curriculum (i.e., using food labels, MyPyramid, accepting body size differences).[1,2]			

Local Wellness Policy (LWP) Checklist (Continued).

State:			**District Contact Name:**	
School District:			**Contact Information:**	
		Addressed in Policy	**Not Addressed in Policy**	**Note**
	Nutrition education instruction by specific teacher type (i.e., classroom teacher, health teacher, school nurse).[1]			
	Nutrition education as part of other classes in addition to health education.[1]			
	Mention of specific number of contact hours for nutrition education.[1]			
	Nutrition education training for teachers and other staff.[1,2]			
	Other:			
Nutrition Guidelines				
	Meals served through the National School Lunch and Breakfast Programs meet, at a minimum, nutrition requirements established by USDA, State, or district policies.			
	Agreements with food or vending companies to sell foods or beverages in schools shall ensure that contractors follow the district's nutritional standards.[1]			
	Food and beverages sold in cafeterias, vending machines, and school stores meet district's nutrition standards.[1,2]			

	Cut-off points for permissible foods sold individually (i.e., total grams of fat, percentage of total calories from fat, total grams of added sugars).[1]			
	Restrictions on vending machines themselves, hours of operation, or location.[1]			
	Restrictions or suggestions for fundraising.[1,2]			
	Foods and beverages sold at school-sponsored events outside of the school day meet nutrition standards.[1]			
	Other:			
Nutrition Environment				
	Surroundings for eating (i.e., placement of healthier options on lunch lines, promotion of healthy nutrition choices in the physical setting where kids eat).[1]			
	Mealtimes and scheduling.[1,2]			
	Strategy for persons eligible for free and reduced-price meals.			
	Qualifications of school food service staff.[1]			
	Provide continuing professional development for nutrition professionals.[1]			
	Professional development for food service staff.[1]			
	Prohibits use of food as a reward.[1]			
	Prohibits withholding food as punishment.[1]			
	Other:			

Local Wellness Policy (LWP) Checklist (Continued).

State:			**District Contact Name:**	
School District:			**Contact Information:**	
		Addressed in Policy	**Not Addressed in Policy**	**Note**
Physical Education/Physical Activity				
	Curriculum is based upon national or State physical education standards.			
	Physical education is offered daily (i.e., 150 minutes per week for elementary; 225 for secondary).			
	Integration of physical activity into regular classrooms by teaching subjects through physical activity/movement.			
	Integration of physical activity into regular classrooms by having physical activity breaks.			
	Physical education instructor must be certified, licensed, or endorsed.[1]			
	Will not allow substitution (i.e., participation in band, chorus, ROTC) for meeting the physical education requirement.[1]			
	Engages students in moderate to vigorous activity during at least 50% of physical education class time.[1]			
	Daily recess requirements for elementary school students.[1]			

	Physical activity opportunities available before and after school (i.e., safe routes to school).[1]			
	Physical activity will not be used as punishment (i.e., making students do laps, do push-ups, etc.) for bad behavior in any classroom.			
	Physical activity will not be withheld as a punishment.[1]			
	Other:			
Other School-Based Activities That Promote Student Wellness				
	Marketing of food and/or beverages.[3]			
	Access to physical activity facilities.[3]			
	After-school programs.[3]			
	Coordinated school health approach.[3]			
	School health councils.[3]			
	Community/family involvement.[3]			
	Staff wellness.[3]			
	Counseling, psychological, and social health services.[3]			
	Health services.[3]			
	Other:			
	Person identified who willreview policy to ensure compliance.[1]			
	Plan developed to review policy compliance, assess progress, and determine areas in need of improvement.[1]			
	Other:			
District Questions		**Yes**	**No**	**Note**
	Policy includes all required components of the local wellness policy?			

Local Wellness Policy (LWP) Checklist (Continued).

State:			District Contact Name:	
School District:			Contact Information:	
		Addressed in Policy	Not Addressed in Policy	Note
	Policy has been adopted by the school district?			
	Policy was implemented in multiple district schools during 2006-2007?			
	Can these schools be identified?			
	Is the district monitoring implementation of, and adherence to, the policy?			
	District size.			
	Number of schools implementing LWP.			

Source: [1]Schwartz, M.B. (n.d.). *Macro-level predictors of school wellness policies in Connecticut*. Rudd Center for Food Policy and Obesity at Yale University.

[2] California Project LEAN. (2006, October). *Policy in action: A guide to implementing your local school wellness policy* [www.CaliforniaProjectLean.org]. Sacramento, CA: Author.

[3] Action for Healthy Kids. (n.d.). *Wellness Policy Fundamentals*

APPENDIX B. SELECTION CRITERIA: DESCRIPTIONS

Selection Criteria: Descriptions

Potential Impact. The intervention appears to have potential for impact on the social or physical environment pertinent to healthy eating and active living—and ultimately on the target individual behaviors. Potential impact is assessed based on the intervention's conceptual logic and other pertinent characteristics, such as intensity and duration. Estimate of impact is based on "face value," program documents, and brief expert input from funding organization staff and contractors, and other experts who know the intervention but are independent from it.

Innovativeness. Intervention is new or different or a significant variation on an existing promising intervention. Emphasis on innovativeness may be mitigated if the intervention represents a type or category of intervention that is prevalent in the field and/or of particular interest to the Foundation and collaborating organizations.

Reach to Target Population. The likelihood or actual evidence that the intervention will achieve participation (and even retention and completion) by the target population (i.e., approximately what percentage of the target population is likely to or actually does participate in or is "reached" in some other way by the intervention).

Acceptability to Stakeholders. The potential or actual evidence that the intervention is acceptable and even attractive to pertinent collaborators, gatekeepers, and other necessary groups, such as schools, businesses, government agencies, grassroots groups, and so forth.

Feasibility of Implementation. The likelihood that the intervention as designed can be fully implemented given the clarity of its goals, objectives, and strategies; complexity and leadership requirements; financial and other costs; and training and supervision requirements. If evidence exists regarding program implementation, then feasibility refers to the extent to which the intervention "on paper" has been fully and faithfully implemented and the degree of difficulty in achieving implementation.

Feasibility of Adoption. The potential for similar sites or entities to adopt the intervention.

Intervention Sustainability. The likelihood that the intervention can continue over time without special resources or extraordinary leadership.

Generalizability. The degree to which the intervention demonstrates or has potential to be adapted for other populations and settings.

Staff/Organizational Capacity. Sponsoring organization and staff have the capacity to participate fully in a brief assessment, learn from it, and further develop the intervention.

Appendix C. Local Wellness Policy Interview Topics

Local Wellness Policy Interview Topics

During the site visits, we hope to learn more about the local wellness policy in your school district. Some of the topics that we would like to discuss with the identified interviewees include the following:

- **Lead Administrators**
  - Background and history of the policy
  - Development of policy regarding nutrition, physical activity, wellness promotion
  - Prior needs assessment activities and their findings
  - Challenges and barriers to development and implementation of policy
  - Strategies for addressing political, financial, and human resources factors
  - Policy's goals, expected outcomes, activities, and services regarding nutrition, physical activity, wellness promotion
  - Support from the school district and community organizations
  - Administrator's role and responsibilities
  - Profile of community and/or student population
  - Community awareness, involvement, and reaction
  - Policy's reach to target audience
  - Current or potential partnerships
  - Success(es) of the policy
  - Key lessons learned with overall experience
  - Modifications to the policy since its adoption
  - Evaluation plan
  - Data collection of outcomes and data sources
  - Financial resources, funding challenges, future funding mechanisms
  - Startup costs, ratio of costs across policy components, cost of administration
- **Principals**
  - Principal's role in developing and implementing the policy
  - Policy's goals, expected outcomes, activities, and services regarding nutrition, physical activity, wellness promotion

  - Support from the school district and community organizations
  - Challenges and barriers of implementing policy
  - Strategies for addressing political, financial, and human resources factors
  - Profile of community and/or student population
  - Community awareness and involvement
  - Policy's reach to target audience
  - Current or potential partnerships
  - Success(es) of the policy
  - Key lessons learned with overall experience
  - Modifications to the policy since its adoption
  - Evaluation plan
  - Financial resources, funding challenges, and future funding mechanisms
  - Startup costs, ratio of costs across policy components, cost of administration
- **Faculty and Staff**
  - Staff members' role in developing and implementing the policy
  - Policy's goals, expected outcomes, activities, and services regarding nutrition, physical activity, wellness promotion
  - Challenges and barriers of implementing policy
  - Other key staff
  - Profile of community and/or student population
  - Community awareness, involvement, and reaction
  - Policy's reach to target audience
  - Current or potential partnerships
  - Success(es) of the policy
  - Key lessons learned with overall experience
  - Modifications to the policy since its adoption
  - Data collection activities
  - Financial resources, funding challenges, and future funding mechanisms
- **School District Partners in Local Wellness Policy**
  - Partner's involvement, role, and responsibilities in developing and implementing the policy
  - Policy's goals, expected outcomes, activities, and services regarding nutrition, physical activity, wellness promotion
  - Community awareness and involvement

- Challenges of partnership
- Benefits from partnership
- Other potential partners
- Success(es) of the policy
- Key lessons learned from experience with the policy
- Funding sources and their effect on partnership

- **Evaluators**
  - Evaluator's role and responsibilities in developing, implementing, and/or evaluating the policy
  - Policy's goals, expected outcomes, activities, and services regarding nutrition, physical activity, wellness promotion
  - Reach to target audience
  - Community awareness, involvement, and reaction
  - Other potential partners
  - Success(es) of the policy
  - Evaluation design
  - Data collection activities and methods
  - Analysis of data and dissemination of results
  - Key lessons learned from experience with policy and efforts with evaluation
  - Financial resources, funding challenges, and future funding mechanisms
- **Other Stakeholders**
  - Background and history of the policy
- **Policy's goals, expected outcomes, activities, and services regarding nutrition, physical activity, wellness promotion**
  - Stakeholder's role and involvement with the local wellness policy
  - Community awareness, involvement, and reaction
  - Other potential partners
  - General impression of the local wellness policy
  - General impact of specific changes in physical activity or eating behavior
  - Success(es) of the policy
  - Key lessons learned from experience with the policy
  - Knowledge of policy's funding

Appendix D. Local Wellness Policy Logic Model

Local Wellness Policy Logic Model

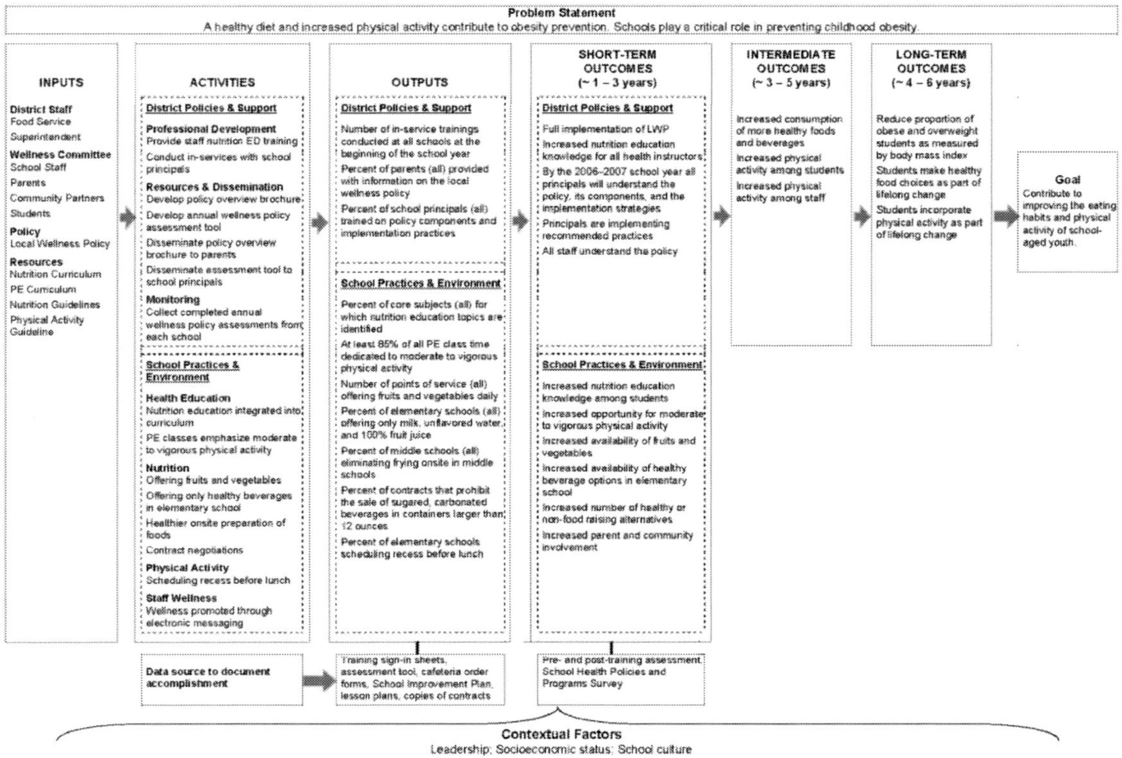

REFERENCES

Adelman, H. S. & Taylor, L. (2005). *The school leader's guide to student learning supports: New directions for addressing barriers to learning*. Thousand Oaks, CA: Corwin Press.

Bergman, E. A., Buergel, N. S., Englund, T. F. & Femrite, A. (2004). The relationship of meal and recess schedules to plate waste in elementary schools. *Journal of Child Nutrition and Management*, *28(8)*, Retrieved June 28, 2008, from http://docs.schoolnutrition.org/newsroom/jcnm/04fall/bergman/bergman1.asp

Bernard, H. R. (2000). *Social research methods: Qualitative and quantitative approaches*. Thousand Oaks, CA: Sage.

Centers for Disease Control and Prevention. (1996). Guidelines for school health programs to promote lifelong healthy eating. *Morbidity and Mortality Weekly Report*, *45(RR-99)*, 1-41.

Centers for Disease Control and Prevention. (1997). Guidelines for school and community programs to promote lifelong physical activity among young people. *Morbidity and Mortality Weekly Report*, *46(RR-6)*, 1-36.

Getlinger, M., Laughlin, C., Bell, E., Akre, C. & Arjmandi, B. (1996). Food waste is reduced when elementary-school children have recess before lunch. *Journal of the American Dietetic Association*, *96*, 906-908.

Gortmaker, S. L., Peterson, K.., Wiecha, J., Sobol, A. M., Dixit, S., Fox, M. K. et al. (1999). Reducing obesity via a school-based interdisciplinary intervention among youth: Planet Health. *Archives of Pediatric and Adolescent Medicine*, *153(4)*, 409-418.

Hedley, A. A., Ogden, C. L., Johnson, C. L., Carroll, M. D., Curtin, L. R. & Flegal, K. M. (2004). Prevalence of overweight and obesity among US children, adolescents, and adults, 1999-2002. *Journal of the American Medical Association*, *291*, 2847-2850.

Hoelscher, D. M., Feldman, H. A., Johnson, C. C., Lytle, L. A., Osganian, S. K., Parcel, G. S. et al. (2004). School-based health education programs can be maintained over time: Results from the CATCH institutional study. *Preventive Medicine*, *38*, 594-606.

Institute of Medicine. (2007). Nutrition standards for foods in schools: *Leading the way toward healthier youth*. Washington, DC: The National Academies Press.

Joint Committee on Health Education and Promotion Terminology. (2001). Report of the 2000 Joint Committee on Health Education and Promotion Terminology. *American Journal of Health Education*, *32(2)*, 89-103.

Joint Committee on National Health Education Standards. (2007). *National Health Education Standards*: Achieving Excellence (2nd Ed.). Atlanta, GA: American Cancer Society.

Lee, S., Burgeson, C. R., Fulton, J. E. & Spain, C. G. (2007). Physical education and physical activity: Results from the School Health Policies and Programs Study 2006. *Journal of School Health*, *77(8)*, 435-463.

National Association for Sport & Physical Education. (2005). Understanding the difference: Is it physical education or physical activity? Reston, VA: Author.

Ogden, C. L., Carroll, M. D. & Flegal, K. M. (2008). High body mass index for age among US children and adolescents, 2003–2006. *Journal of the American Medical Association*, *299*, 2401-2405.

O'Toole, T., Anderson, S., Miller, C. & Guthrie, J. (2007). Nutrition services and foods and beverages available at school: Results from the School Health Policies and Programs Study 2006. *Journal of School Health*, *77(8)*, 500-521.

Patton, M. Q. (1997). Utilization-focused evaluation: The new century text. Thousand Oaks, CA: Sage. Patton, M. Q. (2002). *Qualitative research methods & evaluation methods*. Thousand Oaks, CA: Sage.

Perry, C. L., Stone, E. J., Parcel, G. S., Ellison, R. C., Nader, P. R., Webber, L. S., et al. (1990). School-based cardiovascular health promotion: The child and adolescent trial for cardiovascular health (CATCH). *Journal of School Health*, *60(8)*, 406-413.

U.S. Census Bureau. (2006). Back to School: 2006-2007 (CB06-FF.11-2). Retrieved June 28, 2008, from http://www.census.gov/Press-Release/www/releases/archives/facts_for_features_special_editions/007108.html

U.S. Department of Agriculture. (2004). Executive Summary. Evaluation of the School Breakfast Program Pilot Project. Retrieved June 28, 2008, from
http://www.fns.usda.gov/oane/MENU/Published/CNP/FILES/breakfastyr1.htm

Wechsler, H., McKenna, M. L., Lee, S. M. & Deitz, W. H. (2004). The role of schools in preventing childhood obesity: Childhood obesity. *The State Education Standard*, (4-12).

Wholey, J. S. (2004). Evaluability assessment. In J. S., Wholey, H. P. Hatry, & K. E. Newcomer, *Handbook of practical program evaluation*, (33-62). San Francisco: Jossey-Bass.

In: Prevention of Childhood Obesity ISBN: 978-1-61209-962-0
Editor: Christina V. Mancuso, pp. 139-159

Chapter 4

COMPREHENSIVE SCHOOL PHYSICAL ACTIVITY PROGRAMS

Christina V. Mancuso

ACKNOWLEDGMENTS

This project is a collaborative effort led by a team from the Robert Wood Johnson Foundation (RWJF); the Centers for Disease Control and Prevention's (CDC) Division of Nutrition, Physical Activity and Obesity, Division of Adolescent and School Health, and Division of Adult and Community Health's Prevention Research Centers Program Office; and the CDC Foundation. The project team is advised by the Funder's Advisory Committee, which includes representatives from the RWJF, the National Institutes of Health, the U.S. Department of Agriculture (USDA), WK Kellogg Foundation, and Kaiser Permanente. IFC Macro, an ICF International Company, serves as the coordinating center for the project.

We are grateful to the staff at the school districts for welcoming members of our project team to their sites and allowing us to learn more about their exemplary efforts. It is evident that there is a lot of energy and enthusiasm in the schools as it relates to the implementation of the comprehensive school physical activity program. We applaud the tremendous efforts that schools have put forth in promoting health and wellness among students and staff.

I. Introduction

Background

Early Assessment of Programs and Policies to Prevent Childhood Obesity was a 2-year project to identify and assess local-level programs and policies that have been implemented with apparent success to prevent obesity by improving the eating habits and physical activity levels of children aged 3 to 17 years. In each year of the project, a systematic search process identified programs and policies, and then an expert panel suggested further exploration of the most promising programs and policies. Priority was given to programs and policies that addressed low-income populations and ethnic groups with disproportionate childhood obesity.

Purpose of Early Assessment

As the search for answers to effectively address childhood obesity continues, organizations and communities across the country are experimenting with various strategies aimed at changing children's environments to prevent obesity. The Systematic Screening and Assessment (SSA) Method is a new evaluation approach to identify and assess several innovations being implemented in the field within a relatively short period of time. Innovations are assessed both for their potential impact on health outcomes and their readiness for evaluation.

As part of the SSA Method, evaluability assessments were used to assess the plausibility and feasibility of selected programs and policies that were identified as promising during the search process and selected by the project's expert panel. Evaluability assessment is a process in which evaluators work with program administrators and stakeholders to determine an initiative's readiness for evaluation (Patton, 1997). It involves clarifying goals and program design by specifying the program model, determining stakeholders' views on the important issues, and exploring program reality (Wholey, 2004). Evaluability assessments can help determine whether a rigorous evaluation study (e.g., an experimental evaluation such as a randomized control trial) is feasible and merited for a particular program or policy. As such, they can help avoid premature investment in rigorous evaluation of programs or policies that have not been adequately implemented and allow evaluation resources to be targeted to programs or policies deemed ready for rigorous evaluation.

Focus Areas

During the second year of the project, the Funder's Advisory Committee identified four thematic areas: child care programs and policies in afterschool and day care settings, programs or policies increasing access to healthier foods, comprehensive school physical activity programs, and the built environment.

This synthesis report focuses on the evaluability assessments conducted on comprehensive school physical activity (CSPA) programs. CSPA programs encompass programming before, during, and after the school day (National Association for Sport and Physical Education, 2008). These programs are implemented in elementary, middle, and high schools and provide physical activity opportunities for all students. Goals of the program are to provide physical activity opportunities that enable students to accumulate a total of 60 minutes of physical activity per day. NASPE recommends that a CSPA program include: quality physical education; school-based physical activity opportunities; school employee wellness and involvement; and family and community involvement. Physical activity opportunities can include recess, physical activity breaks and movement during instruction, intramurals or physical activity clubs, interscholastic sports, and walk and bike to school initiatives (National Association for Sport and Physical Education, 2005).

This report describes the extent to which CSPA programs have been implemented and the limitations of implementation in one school and one school district. The report concludes with lessons learned and recommendations to inform future implementation by district and school personnel and other key decision makers.

Relevant Literature

Among children aged 6 to 11 years, 33.3% are overweight or obese; among adolescents aged 12 to 19 years, 34.1% are overweight or obese (Ogden, Carroll, & Flegal, 2008). Physical inactivity is one of the leading causes of childhood obesity (Wang, Gortmaker, Sobol, & Kuntz, 2006). With millions of children and adolescents enrolled, schools play a critical role in making physical activity possible through quality physical education and other school-based opportunities (Wechsler, McKenna, Lee, & Dietz, 2004). According to the 2007 Youth Risk Behavior Survey, only 34.7% of students reported being physically active for a total of at least 60 minutes per day on 5 or more days per week (Eaton et al., 2008). The U.S. Dietary Guidelines for Americans recommend that young people (aged 6 to 19) participate in at least 60 minutes of physical activity daily (U.S. Department of Health and Human Services & U.S. Department of Agriculture, 2005). For this reason, the Centers for Disease Control and Prevention (CDC) and the National Association for Sport and Physical Education (NASPE) recommend a comprehensive approach to enhancing physical education and physical activity in schools to increase students' engagement in physical activity (Lee, Burgeson, Fulton, & Spain, 2007; National Association for Sport and Physical Education, 2008).

II. METHODS

Nomination of Programs

The project team solicited nominations for CSPA programs between September and October 2007 from schools and districts across the United States through postings on a variety of listservs (e.g., the Comprehensive Health Education Network) and through direct contact with the CDC's Division of Adolescent and School Health project officers and funded school health program coordinators. Nominated programs were eligible for inclusion in the project if the program: (1) was a school-based physical activity program; (2) provided the opportunity for students to engage in at least 30 minutes of moderate to vigorous physical activity during each school day (when combined with activity in physical education class to equal at least 60 minutes of physical activity); (3) promoted physical activity opportunities to and/or included ALL students; (4) included a physical education component that offered instruction at least 3 days per week; (5) included a written curriculum; (6) had physical education standards that were consistent with national and/or State standards for physical education; (7) prohibited waivers or exemptions for participation in other school- or community-sponsored activities; (8) offered at least two of the following physical activity strategies: recess for elementary school students, physical activity breaks and movement during instruction, intramurals or physical activity clubs, or walk and bike to school initiatives; (9) offered interscholastic sports at the middle or high school level; (10) had been in existence for more than 6 months; and (11) had not been rigorously evaluated. A total of 30 programs were nominated; 7 met our criteria for inclusion and were reviewed by the expert panel.

Criteria and Selection of Programs for Evaluability Assessments

We convened a panel of 15 experts in evaluation, measurement, physical activity, school-aged youth, and community programs in January 2008. Specific criteria to select programs for evaluability assessment were developed by the project team in collaboration with the expert panel. These criteria included potential impact of the program; innovativeness; reach to target population; acceptability to stakeholders; feasibility of implementation; feasibility of adoption; sustainability; generalizability; and staff and organizational capacity of the implementers (see Appendix A for a detailed description of each criterion). The expert panel reviewed summaries of each of the seven comprehensive school physical activity programs, scored each program on each criterion through an Internet-based survey tool, and made recommendations on which programs would receive evaluability assessments. After each panel member scored each policy and discussed each program as a group, four CSPA programs were recommended for evaluability assessments (EA). The expert panel recommended three programs be combined into a cluster EA with a single site visit because they were a part of the same district and shared many program components. The panel recommended a total of two evaluability assessments.

Comprehensive School Physical Activity Program Evaluability Assessments

Each EA involved (1) a review of background documentation about the program; (2) the development of a program logic model to outline program goals and activities; and (3) a 2.5-day site visit, in which trained site visitors assessed implementation, data collection, and evaluation capacity through interviews with program staff and partners. One school was visited in Washington and one school district was visited in West Virginia. Each evaluability assessment site visit was conducted by two site visitors who traveled to the program. Interviews were conducted with individuals involved with the program, such as school district personnel, principals, physical education teachers, parents, community partners, and other stakeholders. Interview questions addressed program development, implementation, evaluation, and funding (see Appendix B for the full list of interview topics). The project team and expert panel reviewed the findings from all the evaluability assessments to determine the degree of promise of the programs and their readiness for rigorous evaluation.

Data Analysis

Site visit reports were created from each site visit and were the primary data sources for this synthesis report. Reports were analyzed for themes using open coding of qualitative data (Bernard, 2000). Three team members initially identified codes in the texts of the site visit reports. Each individual developed codes independently after reviewing the site visit reports, then compared and discussed similarities and differences to arrive at a single comprehensive list of codes for analysis (Patton, 2002). One team member then coded all reports from each site. ATLAS.ti (version 5.0) was used to categorize and sort data within codes. Secondary data sources included expert panel preliminary review perspectives and expert panel post-site visit recommendations. Site visitors have reviewed a draft of the results section of this report for accuracy of interpretation.

III. BACKGROUND

Setting Characteristics

The two sites selected to receive an evaluability assessment included one high school in Washington with 6,339 students and one school district in West Virginia with 13,519 students. These two school settings, both rural, served a majority White student population with free and reduced-price lunch rates that were below 50% (18% in Washington and 40% in West Virginia).

Development of Programs

The two CSPA programs are longstanding. The high school CSPA program in Washington was created in 1997 with quality physical education as the cornerstone with the addition of various physical activity opportunities for students and staff over time. Three physical education teachers created and still run the program. In West Virginia, their CSPA program is part of a larger district-wide health initiative. The larger district-wide health initiative began out of a concern regarding overweight and cardiovascular risk factors among students in the county. Health screenings were the initial component of the program, followed by various healthy lifestyle interventions. The CSPA program is one component of this larger initiative that focuses on physical activity. The initiative was created and is still headed by a dedicated director.

Goals and Outcomes of CSPA Programs

The primary goals of both CSPA programs are to encourage physical activity at school, provide students with the necessary skills to engage in proper physical activity, and expose students to a variety of physical activity opportunities to find activities they enjoy. Expected outcomes of both programs included: meeting state physical education standards; increased opportunities for physical activity; increased knowledge, attitudes, motor skills, and confidence needed to adopt and maintain physically active lifestyles among students; improved performance; development of lifetime activity skills and interests; and increased student time engaged in moderate and vigorous activity overall (in and out of school).

Target Audience

The primary target audience for the comprehensive school physical activity programs is all students enrolled in the high school in Washington and all elementary school students in the district in West Virginia.

IV. Logic Model

As part of the EAs, each program developed a logic model describing inputs and activities and outputs. An example of a logic model is provided in Appendix C. The following section describes a) inputs and b) activities and outputs from each of the two programs.

Inputs

Funding

Outside of physical education teacher salaries (which are paid by the district in both sites), funding sources varied for each program. At the high school in Washington, the annual physical education department budget was set by the school and ranged from \$5,000 to \$7,000 annually. It was expected that there would be a 10% decrease in the 2008–2009 budget. In West Virginia, however, their larger district-wide health initiative, of which CSPA is a part, was funded primarily through grants totaling more than \$700,000 over the life of the initiative, which began in 2001. It was not clear how much of this funding was dedicated to CSPA or to schools specifically for its implementation; however, funding was not used to support teacher time directly.

Staffing

The two CSPA programs were staffed with qualified physical education teachers, who regularly engaged in physical education professional development. Both programs considered physical education understaffed for the number of students enrolled. For example, at the high school two- thirds of the student population (approximately 650) enrolled in daily physical education classes with three physical education teachers. Due to the large class sizes (i.e., 40 to 45 students), the daily 2-year physical education requirement and interest from students in physical education, a need for additional physical education teachers exists at the high school in Washington. As a result, limited opportunities are available before and after school because staff are overwhelmed by their physical education classes and additional responsibilities. In fact, the ability to offer opportunities for physical activity outside of the traditional school day is at the discretion of the physical education staff.

Activities and Outputs

Physical Education

Quality physical education is the cornerstone of both CSPA programs. At the high school in Washington, 2 years of physical education is required for graduation, and is offered on a daily basis for 50 minutes. The physical education courses in the high school emphasized "lifetime" activities, which include types of physical activities that adults engage in, such as weight training, dance, golf, and tennis. Physical education courses also focused on improving performance, in accordance with F.I.T.T.R (frequency, intensity, type, time, and reversibility), which is a basic philosophy of what is necessary to gain a training effect from an exercise program. The high school offered a variety of options for physical education, including freshman-year physical education that is required and treated as an "exposure" year to a variety of lifetime sport and activities, focusing on the basic skills needed to enjoy various physical activities for a lifetime (e.g., how to train for a marathon). Upper- level, elective physical education courses allowed students to "specialize" in activities that interest them. In addition, every effort was made to increase participation in physical education through courses like Zero-hour PE, which was offered 1 hour before the school day began, and Saturday PE, which was offered on Saturday mornings. Both classes allowed students with full schedules, as well as any interested student, to participate in physical education class outside the regular school day.

At elementary schools, district-wide in West Virginia, the availability of physical education classes varied, with schools providing at least 90 minutes of structured physical education per week (three times per week). Two schools were successful in increasing their physical education class minutes because the 6th grade classes moved to the middle school. At the time of the site visit, the district was using grant funding to work with middle schools to increase physical education from one semester to a full year (initially, the total amount of physical education minutes would be spread out over the course of the school year, rather than compressed in a single semester). Although the amount of time for physical education would not be increased, classes would be spaced in a way to extend over the year. This process has been very challenging due to space and class schedule constraints.

In both CSPA programs, professional development, supported by the school district, is a top priority for implementing a quality program. In Washington, physical education teachers engaged in ongoing physical education training. In addition, the district has facilitated curriculum alignment for physical education to ensure that all physical education classes met the appropriate standards. West Virginia, with funding from the Carol M. White Physical Education Program Grant, offered numerous physical education and physical activity workshops for physical education teachers and classroom teachers. This district demonstrated an interest in ensuring all instructors received training in physical activity. For example, action-based learning trainings were conducted with physical education teachers, school nurses, health educators, and classroom teachers. In addition, the district created a professional development opportunity that allowed physical education teachers across the district to share ideas for instruction in physical education with each other, in partnership with a local university. In an effort to raise the level of physical education to that of core subjects, the district supported the development of a white book which outlined physical education requirements for each grade (pre-K through 12). The focus shifted from one of sports to one of life skills.

School-Based Physical Activity Opportunities

In addition to physical education, these CSPA programs have implemented school-based physical activities to increase the amount of physical activity kids engaged in. In West Virginia, recess was available to all students for 15 to 20 minutes daily at the elementary school level. In some cases, teachers took students out in the afternoon for a second recess. Other elementary school activities included: dances, action-based learning activities, 1-mile walks, and brain break activities. In one school, grant funding was used to purchase a bag of physical activity equipment for each classroom teacher to use on the playground.

Elementary schools also sponsored physical activity events during the school day. For example, one school hosted a physical education day where students in each grade took turns doing a range of activities focused on fitness and eating right and were awarded prizes. Another school sponsored "Relay for Life" for 2 years that promoted physical activity. Other schools have also sponsored "turn off the television" challenges to promote physical activity and awarded prizes.

Both CSPA programs also provided faculty and staff fitness opportunities. For example, faculty and staff were able to use athletic equipment at school. In addition, physical activity promotion activities for staff included Biggest Loser contests and providing incentives such as pedometers.

School facilities were also open to the community. For example, West Virginia community members used the gymnasiums during the evenings and on weekends. Walking tracks, fields, and playgrounds are also used by the community.

Family- and Community-Oriented Physical Activities

Each CSPA program made an effort to promote physical activity for family and community members. In West Virginia, the district offered $500 mini-grants to parent-teacher associations to organize family events promoting physical activity. The schools visited during the site visit hosted family events multiple times throughout the year (e.g., poster contests, Dance Revolution exhibits, skating rink events, and bowling). One school's physical education teacher also maintained a Web site where families could access MyPyramid or the American Heart Association's Web site for additional information on physical activity. Another physical education teacher occasionally sent home calendars that noted physical activities families could do together all month long. In Washington, a number of community organizations, including the local Parks and Recreation Department, offered intramural sports opportunities to high school students and these activities were strongly supported by the community.

V. EVALUATION ACTIVITIES

Although conducting evaluation is not a formal component of these CSPA programs, program administrators were strongly interested in better understanding the impact of their CSPA program on students. At the high school in Washington, all three physical education teachers were interested in evaluation. They were particularly interested in answering the following questions: What is the potential impact of the program after graduation? Is the high school doing the right thing in terms of course offerings? What do parents think of the program? What are the long-term outcomes of the physical education program on students? How is academic success affected by their quality physical education program?

In West Virginia, schools collected some data including: height, weight, and blood pressure as part of annual health screenings. In addition, they conducted screenings for Acanthosis nigricans (a brown to black velvety hyperpigmentation of the skin caused by elevated level of insulin and associated with obesity and diabetes mellitus), collected data on activity levels from random samples of students, and surveyed students on how active they were in physical education class. They also documented changes in physical activity in classrooms through surveys.

Both CSPA programs lacked sufficient staff and resources to carry out a comprehensive evaluation of their CSPA program. In West Virginia, the district partnered with the director of the Department of Public Health and a faculty member at a local university to conduct some evaluation. The high school in Washington was considering partnering with a local university to assist with evaluation. With this support for evaluation and additional funding, these programs could have the capacity to conduct a comprehensive evaluation.

VI. DISCUSSION

Plausibility

Comprehensive school physical activity programs are built on scientific evidence that supports students being active for at least 60 minutes per day as one strategy to prevent childhood obesity (National Association for Sport and Physical Education, 2008). The CSPA programs in West Virginia and Washington are great examples of programs that seek to provide all kids with multiple opportunities to engage in physical activity during the school day. Physical education is one component of the program that appeared to be implemented systematically for both programs. In both programs, physical education was taught by teachers who were certified and engaged in ongoing professional development. In addition, physical education classes in both programs were filled with movement, activity, and creativity. The amount of physical education class time was a challenge for West Virginia's program, in which the amount of physical education fell short of meeting national recommendations of 150 minutes of physical education per week (National Association for Sport and Physical Education, 2001), even though it met State requirements (90 minutes per week). Administrators for both programs recognize the benefit of solid physical education and continue to strive to improve what is made available to students. In addition, schools make a variety of physical activity opportunities available for students, drawing on the experience, creativity, knowledge, and training of school staff. Teachers make a concerted effort to reach all students with school-based physical activities, striving to attain 60 minutes of physical activity, which is challenging. If both programs were expanded to systematically include a broad range of opportunities outside of physical education, they could supplement current efforts to increase physical activity among students. Coupled with proper nutrition, physical activity is a key piece of the equation in preventing obesity through comprehensive obesity prevention programs in schools.

Feasibility

The CSPA programs in West Virginia and Washington currently include physical education and various school-based opportunities for physical activity. Support for implementation of these programs is provided through multiple opportunities: collaboration among physical education teachers and other classroom teachers, available professional development, and willing district and school administrators. Both programs take advantage of opportunities to continue to add physical activity to the school day through integrative learning, before-school activities, and active physical education classes. The lack of a strategic plan for both programs, however, limits their ability to determine if both programs are being implemented fully. Implementation is limited by current challenges within the school system including meeting national standards for physical education which faces challenges due to insufficient staff, scheduling, space, and time constraints. In addition, both programs benefit greatly from the commitment school personnel make to providing physical activity opportunities outside of physical education. These activities, although limited, are products of the willingness and creativity of dedicated staff. Full implementation in these and other school settings is possible but would need a strategic plan, strong administrative support, financial support, and dedicated staff to fully implement a CSPA program.

VII. Key Lessons Learned

Key lessons were learned about the implementation of CSPA programs through the evaluability assessments. These lessons are outlined below. See Table 1 in Appendix B for recommendations.

- CSPA programs require one or more physical activity champions at the district and school levels to identify the physical activity needs and to support building-level implementation.
- A strong commitment from administrators for quality physical education is critical. Because of the challenges of staff, space, and time constraints, a commitment from administrators ensures that physical education is a priority.
- Funding is critical for CSPA programs. Funding is not only needed for physical education, but particularly for opportunities for physical activity outside of physical education.
- A quality physical education program needs to be the cornerstone of any school-based program. It allows students to learn the necessary skills to engage in physical activity.
- Physical activities before, during, and after school need to be implemented regularly and systematically to impact all students.
- Maximizing use of outdoor space (e.g., walking trails, play equipment, playgrounds) increases opportunities for physical activity not only for students and staff, but also for community members.
- Schools and CSPA programs greatly benefit from collaborations with community organizations that are able to provide opportunities and resources for physical activity.
- Physical activity professional development is essential for both physical education teachers and traditional classroom teachers.
- CSPA programs would benefit from using the Physical Education Curriculum Analysis Tool to analyze physical education curricula (Centers for Disease Control and Prevention, 2006).

- More physical activities need to be targeted toward staff to encourage positive role modeling.
- State Departments of Education need to provide support through policies to ensure that districts and schools provide sufficient time for daily physical education and professional development and technical assistance in developing comprehensive school physical activity programs.
- Regular monitoring and evaluation are necessary to identify ways to improve CSPA programs.

VIII. Conclusion

Comprehensive school physical activity is still a relatively new concept, and these programs have the potential to significantly impact the health of youth attending school. However, CSPA programs require support beyond physical education. State and district support is needed to implement a broad range of activities before, during, and after school. In addition, financial resources are necessary to adopt curricula, hire certified physical education teachers, and promote school-based physical activity. Furthermore, policies are critical to creating a culture of physical activity in schools. If these steps are taken, schools can fully implement comprehensive programs that promote physical activity throughout the entire school day.

Appendix A. Description of Selection Criteria

Description of Selection Criteria

Potential Impact. The intervention may affect the social or physical environment pertinent to healthy eating and active living—changing an individual's behavior. Potential impact is assessed based on the intervention's conceptual logic and other pertinent characteristics, such as intensity and duration. Estimate of impact is based on "face value," program documents, and brief expert input from funding organization staff and contractors, and other experts who know the intervention but are independent from it.

Innovativeness. The intervention is new, different, or a significant variation of an existing intervention. Emphasis on innovativeness may be mitigated if the intervention represents an intervention type or category that is prevalent or of particular interest to the group and collaborating organizations.

Reach to Target Population. The likelihood or actual evidence that the intervention will achieve participation (and even retention and completion) by the target population (i.e., approximately what percentage of the target population is likely to or actually does participate in or is "reached" in some other way by the intervention).

Acceptability to Stakeholders. The potential or actual evidence that the intervention is acceptable and even attractive to pertinent collaborators, gatekeepers, and other necessary groups, such as schools, businesses, government agencies, and grassroots groups.

Feasibility of Implementation. The likelihood that the intervention as designed can be fully implemented given the clarity of its goals, objectives, and strategies; complexity and leadership requirements; financial and other costs; and training and supervision requirements. If evidence exists regarding program implementation, then feasibility refers to the intervention "on paper" has been fully and faithfully implemented and the degree of difficulty in achieving implementation.

Feasibility of Adoption. The potential for similar sites or entities to adopt the intervention.

Intervention Sustainability. The likelihood that the intervention can continue over time without special resources or extraordinary leadership.

Generalizability. The degree to which the intervention demonstrates or has potential to be adapted for other populations and settings.

Staff/Organizational Capacity. Sponsoring organization and staff have the capacity to participate fully in a brief assessment, learn from it, and further develop the intervention.

Appendix B. Local Wellness Policy Interview Topics

Local Wellness Policy Interview Topics

During the site visits, we hope to learn more about the local wellness policy in your school district. Some of the topics that we would like to discuss with the identified interviewees include the following:

Lead Administrators

- Background and history of the policy
- Development of policy regarding nutrition, physical activity, wellness promotion
- Prior needs assessment activities and their findings
- Challenges and barriers to development and implementation of policy
- Strategies for addressing political, financial, and human resources factors
- Policy's goals, expected outcomes, activities, and services regarding nutrition, physical activity, and wellness promotion
- Support from the school district and community organizations
- Administrator's role and responsibilities
- Profile of community and student population
- Community awareness, involvement, and reaction
- Policy's reach to target audience
- Current or potential partnerships
- Policy success(es)
- Key lessons learned with overall experience
- Modifications to the policy since its adoption
- Evaluation plan
- Data collection, outcomes, and data sources
- Financial resources, funding challenges, and future funding mechanisms
- Startup costs, ratio of costs across policy components, and cost of administration

Principals

- Principals' role in developing and implementing the policy
- Policy's goals, expected outcomes, activities, and services regarding nutrition, physical activity, and wellness promotion
- Support from the school district and community organizations
- Challenges and barriers of implementing policy
- Strategies for addressing political, financial, and human resources factors
- Profile of community and student population
- Community awareness and involvement
- Policy's reach to target audience
- Current or potential partnerships
- Success(es) of the policy
- Key lessons learned with overall experience
- Modifications to the policy since its adoption
- Evaluation plan
- Financial resources, funding challenges, and future funding mechanisms
- Startup costs, ratio of costs across policy components, and cost of administration

Faculty and Staff

- Staff members' role in developing and implementing the policy
- Policy's goals, expected outcomes, activities, and services regarding nutrition, physical activity, and wellness promotion
- Challenges and barriers of implementing policy
- Other key staff
- Profile of community and student population
- Community awareness, involvement, and reaction
- Policy's reach to target audience
- Current or potential partnerships
- Success(es) of the policy
- Key lessons learned with overall experience
- Modifications to the policy since its adoption
- Data collection activities
- Financial resources, funding challenges, and future funding mechanisms

School District Partners in Local Wellness Policy

- Partners' involvement, role, and responsibilities in developing and implementing the policy
- Policy's goals, expected outcomes, activities, and services regarding nutrition, physical activity, and wellness promotion
- Community awareness and involvement
- Challenges of partnership
- Benefits from partnership
- Other potential partners
- Policy success(es)
- Key lessons learned from experience with the policy
- Funding sources and their effect on partnership

Evaluators

- Evaluators' role and responsibilities in developing, implementing, and evaluating the policy
- Policy's goals, expected outcomes, activities, and services regarding nutrition, physical activity, and wellness promotion
- Reach target audience
- Community awareness, involvement, and reaction
- Other potential partners
- Policy success(es)
- Evaluation design
- Data collection activities and methods
- Data analysis and results dissemination
- Key lessons learned from experience with policy and evaluation efforts
- Financial resources, funding challenges, and future funding mechanisms

Other Stakeholders

- Background and history of the policy
- Policy's goals, expected outcomes, activities, and services regarding nutrition, physical activity, and wellness promotion

- Stakeholders' role and involvement with the local wellness policy
- Community awareness, involvement, and reaction
- Other potential partners
- General impression of the local wellness policy
- General impact of specific changes in physical activity or eating behavior
- Policy success(es)
- Key lessons learned from policy experience
- Knowledge of policy's funding

Table 1. State-, District-, and School-Level CSPA Recommendations.

Districts and schools should:
• Develop a strategic plan to facilitate growth, prioritize activities, and garner support • Increase before- and afterschool opportunities for physical activity district-wide • Identify resources and champions to assist with implementing physical activity • Develop an evaluation plan to systematically monitor and improve implementation • Conduct analysis of physical education curricula using the Physical Education Curriculum Analysis Tool (Centers for Disease Control and Prevention, 2006) • Promote physical activity among staff • Coordinate physical activity for family and community members
States should:
• Assist with policy development to ensure that districts and schools provide sufficient time for daily physical education • Provide support to districts and schools through professional development andtechnical assistance in developing comprehensive school physical activity programs

Appendix C. Comprehensive School Physical Activity Program Logic Model

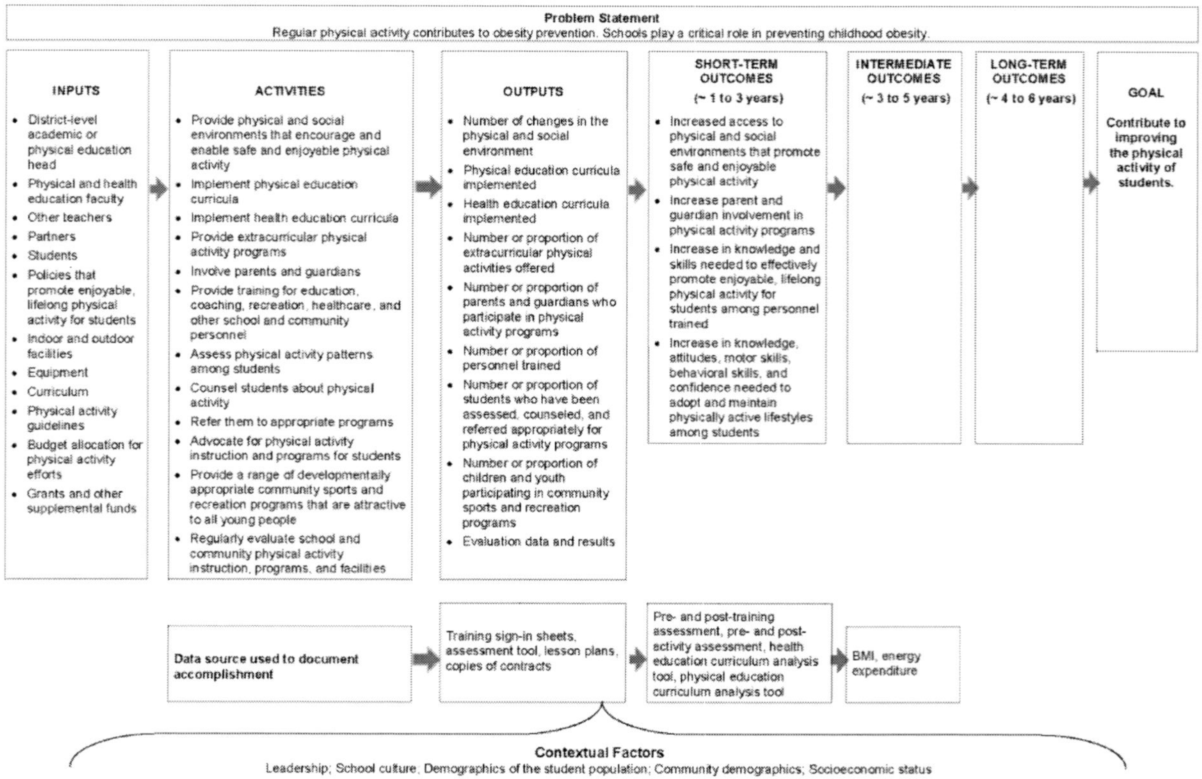

REFERENCES

Bernard, H. R. (2000). *Social research methods: Qualitative and quantitative approaches*. Thousand Oaks, CA: Sage.

Centers for Disease Control and Prevention. (2006). *Physical education curriculum analysis tool*. Atlanta, GA: Author.

Eaton, D., Kann, L., Kinchen, S., Shanklin, S., Ross, J., Hawkins, J., et al. (2008). Youth risk behavior surveillance—United States, 2007. *Morbidity and Mortality Weekly Report, 57(SS-4)*, 1-131.

Lee, S., Burgeson, C., Fulton, J. & Spain, C. (2007). Physical education and physical activity: Results from the School Health Policies and Programs Study 2006. *Journal of School Health, 77(8)*, 435-463.

National Association for Sport and Physical Education. (2001). *Physical education is critical to a complete education*. Reston, VA: Author.

National Association for Sport and Physical Education. (2005). Understanding the difference: Is it physical education or physical activity? *Reston*, VA: Author.

National Association for Sport and Physical Education. (2008). Comprehensive school physical activity programs [Position statement]. *Reston*, VA: Author.

Ogden, C. L., Carroll, M. D. & Flegal, K. M. (2008). High body mass index for age among US children and adolescents, 2003–2006. *Journal of the American Medical Association, 299*, 240 1-2405.

Patton, M. Q. (1997). Utilization-focused evaluation: The new century text. Thousand Oaks, CA: Sage. Patton, M. Q. (2002). *Qualitative research methods & evaluation methods*. Thousand Oaks, CA: Sage.

U.S. Department of Health and Human Services & U.S. Department of Agriculture. (2005). *Dietary guidelines for Americans*, 2005 (6th ed.). Washington, DC: U.S. Government Printing Office.

Wang, Y., Gortmaker, S., Sobol, A. & Kuntz, K. (2006). Estimating the energy gap among U.S. children: A counterfactual approach. *Pediatrics, 118*, 1721-1733.

Wechsler, H., McKenna, M. L., Lee, S. M. & Deitz, W. H. (2004). The role of schools in preventing childhood obesity: Childhood obesity. *The State Education Standard*, (4-12).

Wholey, J. S. (2004). Evaluability assessment. In J. S., Wholey, H. P. Hatry, & K. E. Newcomer, (Eds.), *Handbook of practical program evaluation* (33-62). San Francisco, CA: Jossey-Bass.

Chapter Sources

The following chapters have been previously published:

Chapter 1 – This is an edited, excerpted and augmented edition of a United States Department of Health and Human Services, Centers for Disease Control and Prevention Report dated 2009.

Chapter 2 – This is an edited, excerpted and augmented edition of a United States Department of Health and Human Services, Centers for Disease Control and Prevention Report dated 2009.

Chapter 3 – This is an edited, excerpted and augmented edition of a United States Department of Health and Human Services, Centers for Disease Control and Prevention Report dated 2009.

Chapter 4 – This is an edited, excerpted and augmented edition of a United States Department of Health and Human Services, Centers for Disease Control and Prevention Report dated 2009.

INDEX

A

B

C

D

E

F

G

H

I

Q

R

S

T

U

V

W

Y